THE ULTIMATE GALVESTON DIET COOKBOOK

1500 Days of Nutrient-Rich Recipes to Help You Achieve Your Health Goals and Savor the Flavors of Real Food

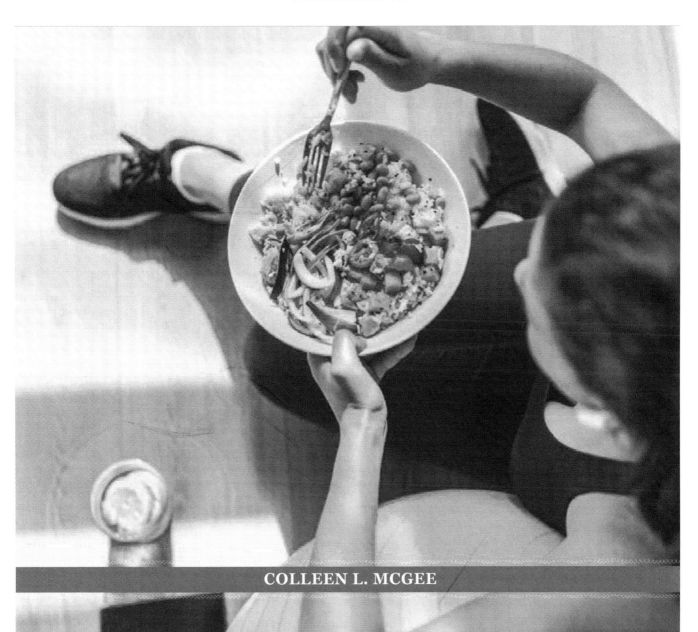

COLLEEN L. MCGEE

EDITOR: LYN

COVER ART: ABR

INTERIOR DESIGN: FAIZAN

FOOD STYLIST: JO

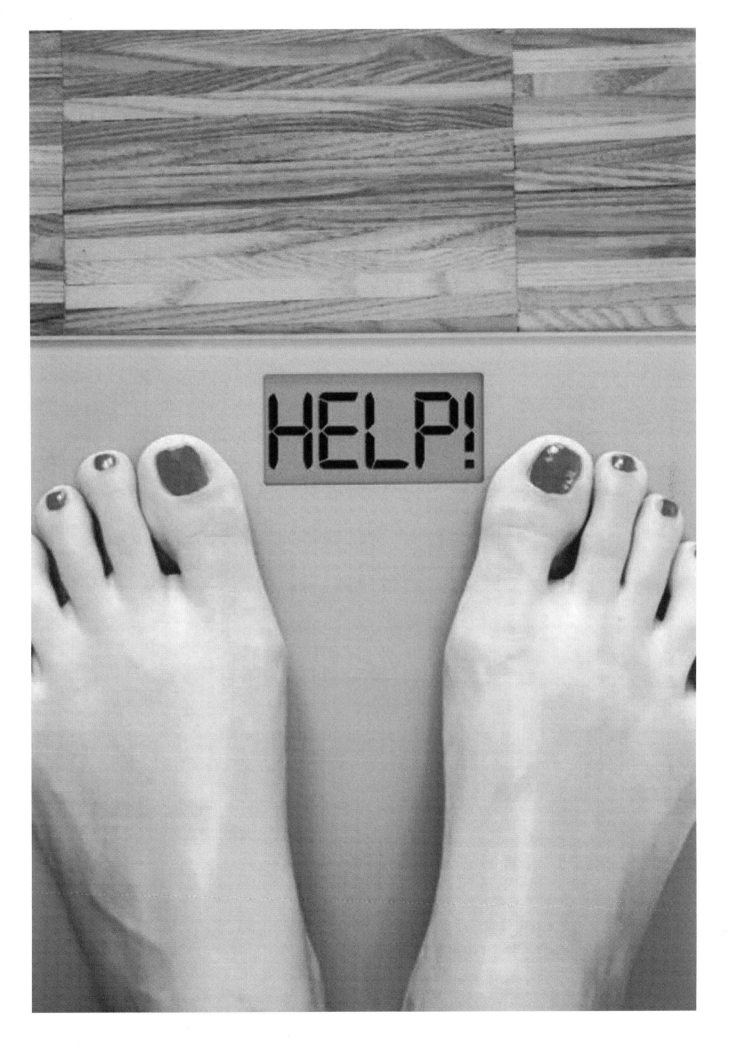

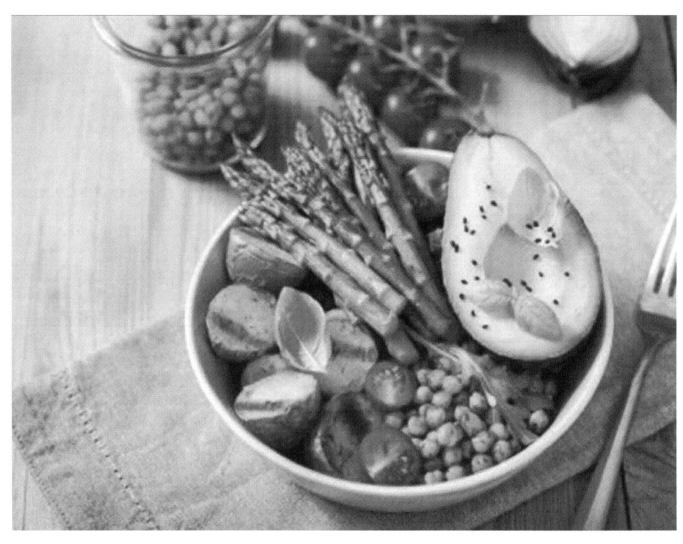

Table of Contents

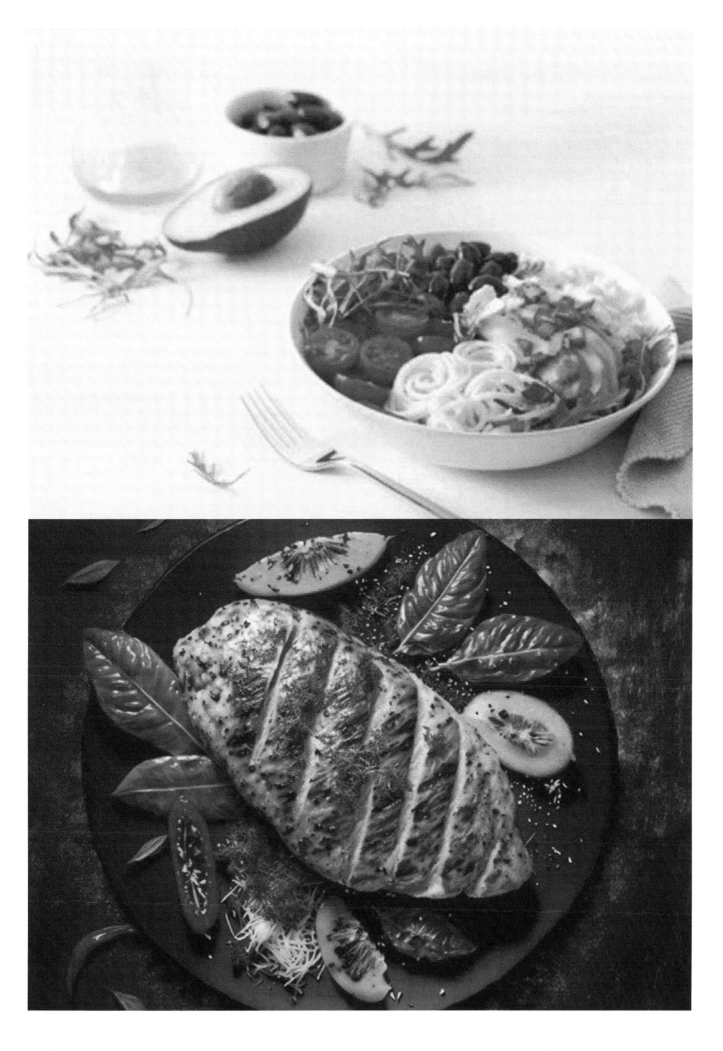

Introduction

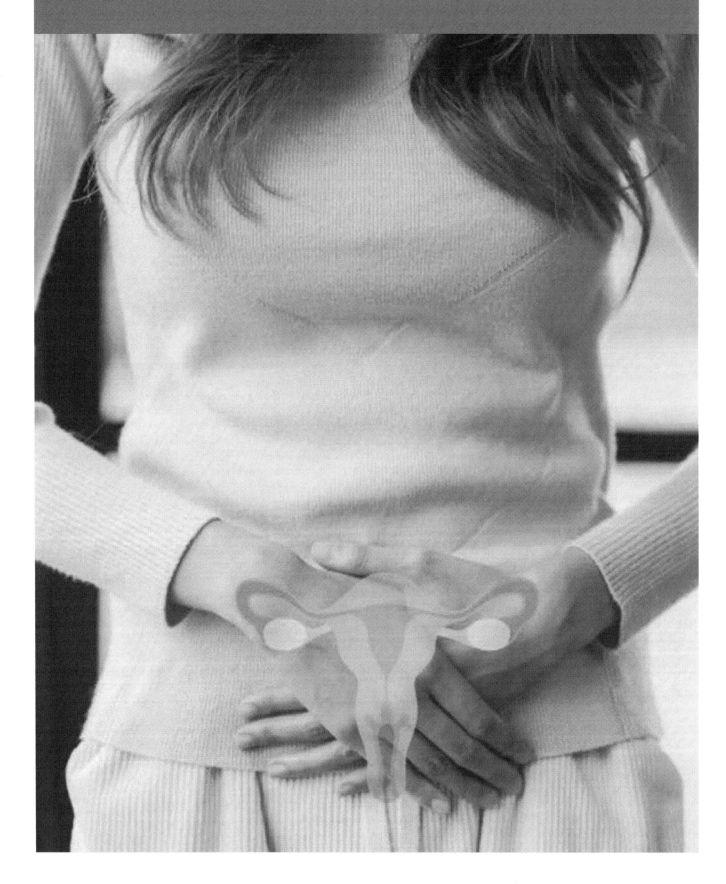

The Galveston Diet is a program that can be especially beneficial for women over 40 years old. As women age, they often experience changes in their bodies that can make it more challenging to lose weight and maintain a healthy lifestyle. However, the Galveston Diet is designed to address many of the issues that women face as they age.

One of the key principles of the Galveston Diet is reducing inflammation in the body. Inflammation can contribute to a range of health problems, including weight gain, joint pain, and fatigue. Women over 40 are more likely to experience inflammation due to hormonal changes and other factors. By following the Galveston Diet, women can reduce inflammation and improve their overall health.

Another important aspect of the Galveston Diet is balancing hormones. As women age, their hormone levels can fluctuate, which can affect their weight, mood, and overall well-being. The Galveston Diet includes foods that can help regulate hormones and promote hormonal balance.

Additionally, the Galveston Diet emphasizes the importance of gut health. The gut is a crucial part of the body's immune system and can affect everything from digestion to mood. Women over 40 may be more likely to experience digestive issues, such as bloating and constipation. By following the Galveston Diet, women can promote a healthy gut and improve their overall digestive health.

Overall, the Galveston Diet can be an excellent program for women over 40 who want to improve their health and lose weight. By reducing inflammation, balancing hormones, and promoting gut health, the Galveston Diet addresses many of the unique challenges that women face as they age. With the support of this program, women can achieve their health and wellness goals and feel their best at any age.

Chapter 1
Understanding the Galveston Diet

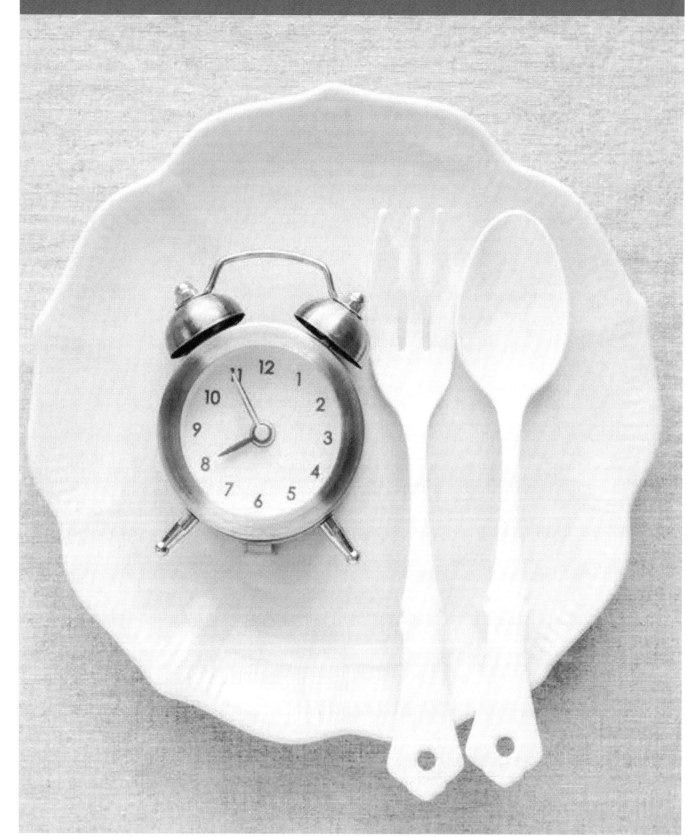

Your Changing Body

The Galveston Diet is specifically designed to address the hormonal changes and challenges that women face as they age, particularly during perimenopause, menopause, and postmenopause.

Perimenopause is a transitional period that usually begins in a woman's late 30s or early 40s. During this time, the body's production of estrogen and progesterone begins to fluctuate, which can cause a variety of symptoms such as irregular periods, hot flashes, night sweats, and mood changes. Perimenopause can last for several years before menopause occurs.

During perimenopause, women experience a gradual decline in estrogen production and fluctuations in other hormones like progesterone. This can cause a range of symptoms such as irregular periods, hot flashes, mood changes, vaginal dryness, and decreased libido.

Menopause is defined as the point in time when a woman has not had a menstrual period for 12 consecutive months. It typically occurs between the ages of 45 and 55, but can happen earlier or later. Menopause marks the end of a woman's reproductive years, as the ovaries no longer release eggs and estrogen production decreases significantly. Symptoms of menopause can include hot flashes, vaginal dryness, sleep disturbances, and mood changes.

Postmenopause refers to the years after menopause, when a woman's hormone levels have stabilized at a lower level. Symptoms of menopause may gradually decrease during this time, but some women may still experience symptoms such as hot flashes or vaginal dryness. Postmenopausal women are at increased risk for certain health conditions such as osteoporosis and heart disease, which is why it's important to maintain a healthy lifestyle and stay up-to-date with regular health screenings.

The diet focuses on reducing inflammation, balancing hormones, and promoting gut health, which can help alleviate common symptoms such as weight gain, fatigue, mood changes, hot flashes, and disrupted sleep. By incorporating nutrient-dense foods that support hormone production and regulation, women may experience improved overall health and well-being during this transitional period.

Background and History of the Galveston Diet

The Galveston Diet is a weight loss program designed specifically for women over 40. It was created by Dr. Mary Claire Haver, a board-certified gynecologist and obstetrician who noticed that many of her patients were struggling with weight gain and related health issues as they aged. Dr. Haver developed the Galveston Diet as a solution to help women over 40 balance their hormones, reduce inflammation, and achieve sustainable weight loss.

The Galveston Diet is based on the idea that hormonal imbalances, inflammation, and poor gut health can contribute to weight gain and health issues. The program focuses on reducing inflammation by eliminating processed foods, sugar, and other inflammatory foods from the diet, while also incorporating hormone-balancing foods and supplements to support overall health. The program also emphasizes the importance of gut health and the gut-brain connection, encouraging the consumption of prebiotic and probiotic-rich foods to support digestive health and overall well-being.

The Galveston Diet program encourages regular exercise and movement, as well as stress-reduction techniques to support mental and emotional health. It is designed to help women over 40 achieve sustainable weight loss and improve their overall health and well-being through a combination of dietary changes, lifestyle modifications, and hormone-balancing supplements. While the program is specifically designed for women over 40, the principles of the diet can be beneficial for anyone looking to improve their health and lose weight in a healthy, sustainable way.

Key Principles of the Galveston Diet

INTERMITTENT FASTING
Intermittent fasting is a method of restricting food intake for a certain period, followed by a period of eating. The Galveston diet utilizes intermittent fasting to promote weight loss and improve overall health. By limiting the number of hours in which food is consumed, the body is forced to use stored energy (fat) as fuel, which can lead to weight loss. The Galveston diet recommends a 16-hour fasting period, followed by an 8-hour eating period, which is known as the 16:8 method.

ANTI-INFLAMMATORY NUTRITION
Anti-inflammatory nutrition is a key component of the Galveston diet. Chronic inflammation in the body has been linked to a range of health problems, including obesity, heart disease, and type 2 diabetes. The Galveston

diet emphasizes the consumption of anti-inflammatory foods like leafy greens, berries, fatty fish, and nuts, while reducing the intake of inflammatory foods like processed foods and sugary drinks. By incorporating anti-inflammatory foods into the diet, the body can reduce inflammation and improve overall health.

FUEL REFOCUS

Fuel refocusing is another principle of the Galveston diet. The program encourages the consumption of foods that support hormone production and regulation, such as lean proteins, healthy fats, and fiber-rich fruits and vegetables. By consuming these foods, women can improve their hormone balance, reduce inflammation, and support overall health.

Benefits of the Galveston Diet

WEIGHT LOSS

The Galveston Diet is designed to help women over 40 lose weight by reducing inflammation, balancing hormones, and promoting gut health. By incorporating lean proteins, healthy fats, fiber-rich fruits and vegetables, and whole grains into their diet, women can increase satiety and reduce cravings, which may lead to weight loss over time.

A study published in the Journal of the Academy of Nutrition and Dietetics found that participants who followed a diet similar to the Galveston Diet, which emphasized lean proteins, healthy fats, and fiber-rich fruits and vegetables, experienced significant weight loss and improvements in metabolic health markers like cholesterol levels and blood pressure.

Another study published in the International Journal of Obesity found that participants who followed a diet high in protein, like the Galveston Diet, experienced greater weight loss and fat loss than those who followed a low-protein diet.

In a survey of Galveston Diet users, 77% of respondents reported losing weight while following the program, with an average weight loss of 10-15 pounds in the first month.

The Galveston Diet also emphasizes the importance of reducing inflammation, which has been linked to obesity and weight gain. By consuming anti-inflammatory foods like fatty fish and leafy greens, individuals on the Galveston Diet may be able to reduce inflammation and support weight loss.

IMPROVED ENERGY LEVELS

The Galveston Diet emphasizes the importance of consuming nutrient-dense foods that provide sustained energy throughout the day. By incorporating whole grains, lean proteins, and healthy fats into their diet, women can stabilize blood sugar levels and avoid energy crashes that are often associated with high-carbohydrate, processed foods.

Following the Galveston Diet can potentially improve energy levels. This is because the diet emphasizes whole, nutrient-dense foods that can provide sustained energy throughout the day. Here are some examples of how the Galveston Diet may improve energy levels:

The Galveston Diet encourages the consumption of complex carbohydrates like whole grains and fiber-rich fruits and vegetables. These foods are broken down slowly by the body, providing a steady release of energy throughout the day.

The diet emphasizes the consumption of lean proteins like chicken, fish, and tofu. These foods are important for building and repairing tissues, including muscle tissue, which can help improve overall energy levels.

The Galveston Diet also encourages the consumption of healthy fats like avocado, nuts, and olive oil. These fats are important for supporting brain health and can help improve cognitive function and energy levels.

By promoting gut health through the consumption of probiotic-rich foods like fermented vegetables and kefir, the Galveston Diet may also improve energy levels. A healthy gut is important for proper nutrient absorption and energy production in the body.

BETTER OVERALL HEALTH

The Galveston Diet is focused on promoting overall health and wellness by reducing inflammation, balancing hormones, and supporting gut health. By consuming nutrient-dense foods that are rich in essential vitamins, minerals, and antioxidants, women can support their immune system, reduce the risk of chronic disease, and improve their overall quality of life.

The Galveston Diet is designed to improve overall health and well-being by addressing the root causes of many health issues, including inflammation, hormonal imbalances, and poor gut health. By emphasizing whole, nutrient-dense foods and promoting healthy lifestyle habits, the Galveston Diet can potentially lead to a wide range of health benefits beyond just weight loss.

For example, reducing inflammation in the body through diet can improve a range of health conditions, such as arthritis, asthma, and allergies. Balancing hormones can also have a positive impact on many aspects of health, including mood, energy levels, and sexual function. And promoting gut health can improve digestion, nutrient absorption, and immune function.

By incorporating lean proteins, healthy fats, fiber-rich fruits and vegetables, and whole grains into the diet, and avoiding processed and inflammatory foods, individuals may experience a wide range of health benefits beyond just weight loss, such as increased energy levels, better sleep quality, and improved mental clarity.

REDUCED INFLAMMATION

Chronic inflammation has been linked to a variety of health issues, including heart disease, diabetes, and certain types of cancer. The Galveston Diet emphasizes the consumption of anti-inflammatory foods like leafy greens, berries, fatty fish, and nuts, which can help reduce inflammation and improve overall health.

Leafy greens, such as kale and spinach, are rich in vitamins, minerals, and antioxidants that can help fight inflammation. Berries, such as blueberries and strawberries, are also high in antioxidants and have anti-inflammatory properties. Fatty fish, such as salmon and sardines, are high in omega-3 fatty acids, which can help reduce inflammation and improve heart health. Nuts, such as almonds and walnuts, are rich in healthy fats and antioxidants that can also help reduce inflammation.

By emphasizing the consumption of these types of foods, the Galveston Diet can help individuals improve their overall health and reduce their risk of developing chronic diseases.

BALANCED HORMONES

Hormonal imbalances are common in women over 40, and can contribute to issues like weight gain, mood swings, and fatigue. The Galveston Diet emphasizes the consumption of foods that support hormone production and regulation, such as lean proteins, healthy fats, and fiber-rich fruits and vegetables.

By consuming foods that are high in essential amino acids, healthy fats, and fiber, women can help regulate their hormone levels, which may lead to improved mood, better sleep, and other health benefits. Additionally, the Galveston Diet recommends limiting or avoiding foods that may disrupt hormone balance, such as processed foods, sugary drinks, and alcohol.

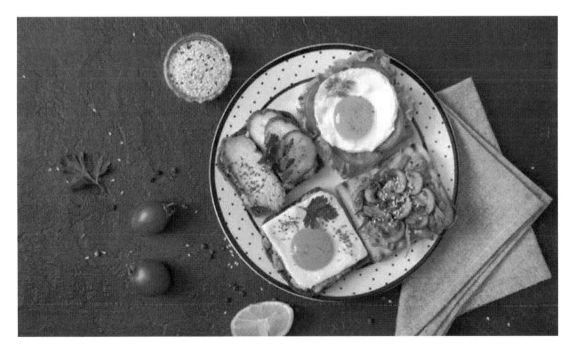

Chapter 2
Start Your Galveston Diet Journey

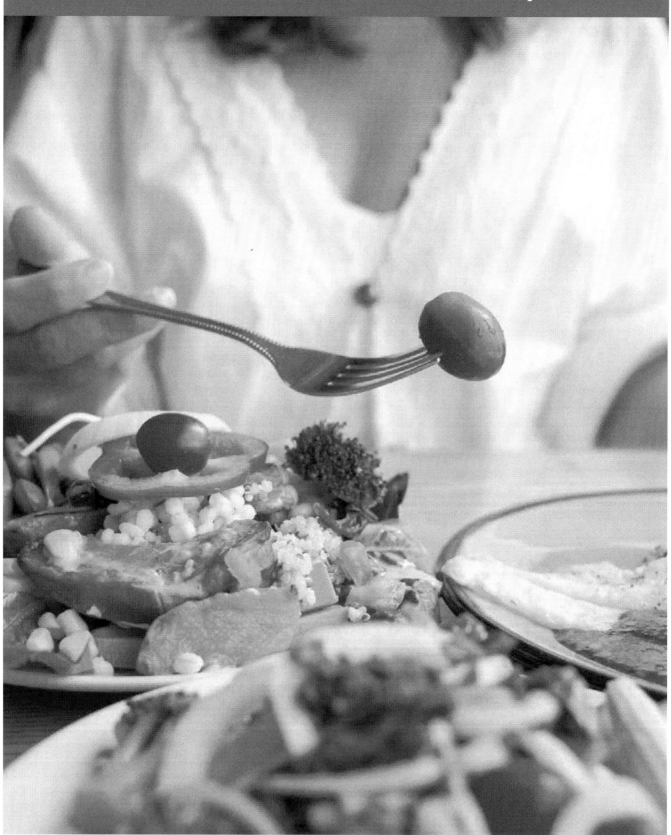

Recommended Foods

LEAN PROTEINS

Protein is an essential nutrient that plays a variety of important roles in the body, including building and repairing tissues, producing enzymes and hormones, and supporting immune function. The Galveston Diet recognizes the importance of protein for overall health and encourages the consumption of lean protein sources that are high in essential amino acids.

Chicken and turkey are popular lean protein sources that are rich in high-quality protein and low in fat. They are also a good source of vitamins and minerals, including B vitamins and selenium. Fish is another lean protein source that is rich in omega-3 fatty acids, which are important for brain and heart health. Eating fish regularly has also been linked to a reduced risk of chronic diseases like heart disease and stroke.

Eggs are a highly nutritious and versatile protein source that are rich in essential amino acids, vitamins, and minerals. They are also a good source of healthy fats, including omega-3 fatty acids, which can help reduce inflammation in the body. Additionally, eggs contain choline, which is important for brain health and may help prevent age-related cognitive decline.

Plant-based protein sources like tofu and beans are also encouraged on the Galveston Diet. Tofu is a good source of plant-based protein that is low in fat and contains all essential amino acids. It is also a good source of iron, calcium, and other important minerals. Beans, such as lentils, chickpeas, and black beans, are also a good source of plant-based protein and are rich in fiber, vitamins, and minerals.

HEALTHY FATS

The Galveston Diet recognizes the importance of healthy fats in the diet and encourages the consumption of foods that are rich in these beneficial fats. Here are some of the reasons why healthy fats are important for overall health and wellness:

1. Regulating hormone production: Hormones play an important role in a variety of bodily processes, including metabolism, mood regulation, and reproductive health. Healthy fats, such as those found in avocados, nuts, and fatty fish, help support the production and regulation of hormones.
2. Promoting satiety: Fats are more calorie-dense than carbohydrates and protein, which means that they can help promote feelings of fullness and satiety. This can help prevent overeating and promote weight loss.
3. Supporting brain health: The brain is composed primarily of fat, and consuming healthy fats is important for maintaining optimal brain function. Omega-3 fatty acids, in particular, are important for brain health and have been linked to a reduced risk of cognitive decline and dementia.
4. Reducing inflammation: Inflammation is a natural response of the immune system to injury or infection, but chronic inflammation can contribute to the development of chronic diseases like heart disease and diabetes. Healthy fats, such as those found in olive oil and nuts, have anti-inflammatory properties and can help reduce inflammation in the body.

Fiber-rich fruits and vegetables

The Galveston Diet encourages the consumption of a wide variety of fruits and vegetables that are rich in fiber, such as leafy greens, berries, broccoli, carrots, and sweet potatoes. These foods are important for promoting gut health, regulating blood sugar levels, and providing essential vitamins and minerals. The Galveston Diet places a strong emphasis on consuming a wide variety of fiber-rich fruits and vegetables, and for good reason. Here are some of the ways that these foods can support overall health and wellness:

1. Promoting gut health: Fiber is important for maintaining a healthy gut microbiome, which is essential for overall digestive health and immune function. Fiber-rich foods, such as leafy greens and broccoli, can help promote the growth of beneficial gut bacteria and reduce the risk of digestive issues like constipation and bloating.
2. Regulating blood sugar levels: High-fiber foods can help regulate blood sugar levels by slowing the absorption of glucose into the bloodstream. This can help prevent spikes in blood sugar and reduce the risk of conditions like type 2 diabetes.
3. Providing essential vitamins and minerals: Fruits and vegetables are excellent sources of essential vitamins and minerals that are important for overall health and wellness. For example, leafy greens are high in vitamin K and folate, while berries are rich in vitamin C and antioxidants.
4. Supporting weight loss: High-fiber foods are often low in calories and can help promote feelings of fullness and satiety. This can make it easier to achieve and maintain a healthy weight.

WHOLE GRAINS

The program recommends incorporating whole grains like quinoa, brown rice, and whole wheat bread into the diet. These foods are high in fiber and important nutrients like B vitamins and iron. Here are some of the ways that these foods can support overall health and wellness:

1. High in fiber: Whole grains are a great source of dietary fiber, which is important for digestive health and can help regulate blood sugar levels. Fiber also promotes feelings of fullness, which can help with weight management.
2. Rich in nutrients: Whole grains are also rich in important nutrients like B vitamins, iron, and magnesium. These nutrients are important for energy production, immune function, and overall health and wellness.
3. May reduce the risk of chronic disease: Consuming whole grains has been associated with a reduced risk of chronic diseases like heart disease, diabetes, and certain types of cancer.
4. Can be a good source of plant-based protein: Some whole grains, like quinoa, are also a good source of plant-based protein. This can be especially beneficial for women over 40 who may need more protein to maintain muscle mass and support overall health.

FERMENTED FOODS

The Galveston Diet emphasizes the importance of incorporating fermented foods into the diet, such as kimchi, sauerkraut, and kefir. These foods are rich in probiotics, which are beneficial bacteria that support gut health. Here are some of the ways that probiotics can support overall health and wellness:

1. Promoting gut health: Probiotics help maintain a healthy balance of bacteria in the gut, which is important for digestive health and immune function. By promoting the growth of beneficial bacteria, probiotics can reduce the risk of digestive issues like bloating and constipation.
2. Supporting immune function: A large portion of the immune system is located in the gut, and probiotics can help support immune function by promoting the growth of beneficial bacteria and reducing the risk of harmful bacteria.
3. Reducing inflammation: Probiotics may help reduce inflammation in the body, which can be beneficial for overall health and wellness. Chronic inflammation has been linked to a variety of health issues, including heart disease, diabetes, and certain types of cancer.
4. May improve mental health: Some research suggests that probiotics may also have a positive impact on mental health by reducing symptoms of anxiety and depression.

Tips for following the Galveston Diet

FIND SUPPORT

Making changes to your diet can be difficult, especially when trying to incorporate new and unfamiliar foods. That's why it's important to have a support system in place to help keep you motivated and on track. One way to do this is to consider joining a Galveston Diet support group or finding online communities of individuals who are also following the program. This can provide a sense of accountability and camaraderie, as well as a source of inspiration and motivation.

Another way to stay motivated is to involve friends and family in your journey. Share your goals with them and ask for their support. You might even consider having a healthy potluck or cooking together to make meal planning and preparation more enjoyable.

Additionally, consider tracking your progress and celebrating your successes along the way. This can help you stay motivated and provide a sense of accomplishment. You might keep a food journal or use a fitness tracker to monitor your progress and set achievable goals for yourself.

Finally, remember that it's okay to make mistakes and slip-ups along the way. Don't let setbacks discourage you from continuing with the Galveston Diet. Instead, use them as opportunities to learn and adjust your approach. With patience, persistence, and a supportive community, you can successfully incorporate the principles of the Galveston Diet into your daily life and achieve your health and wellness goals.

FOCUS ON PROGRESS, NOT PERFECTION

It's completely normal to slip up or struggle when making dietary changes, and it's important to approach the Galveston Diet with a mindset of progress rather than perfection. Recognize that making lasting changes to your eating habits is a process that takes time, patience, and consistency. Don't let a setback discourage you from continuing to make positive changes.

Instead of focusing on being perfect, focus on progress and celebrate small victories along the way. Maybe you were able to stick to the diet for a full week, or you were able to resist a temptation that would have derailed you in the past. Recognizing and celebrating these small wins can help keep you motivated and feeling good about your progress.

It's also helpful to be kind to yourself and practice self-compassion. Instead of criticizing yourself for slip-ups, try to approach them with curiosity and a willingness to learn. Ask yourself what triggered the slip-up and how you can better prepare for similar situations in the future. Remember that setbacks are a natural part of the process, and that progress, not perfection, is the goal.

BE MINDFUL OF PORTION SIZES

In addition to making healthy food choices, portion control is a key component of the Galveston Diet. It's easy to overeat, even when eating healthy foods. Consuming too many calories can stall weight loss progress and lead to weight gain.

Using measuring cups, a food scale, or even visual cues can help you keep portions in check. For example, a serving of meat should be about the size of a deck of cards, while a serving of vegetables should be about the size of your fist. Be mindful of calorie-dense foods like nuts and avocado, and aim to include them in appropriate portions as part of a balanced meal.

By practicing portion control, you can ensure that you're consuming appropriate amounts of food to support your weight loss goals while also getting the nutrients your body needs to function optimally.

STAY HYDRATED

Staying hydrated is essential for many bodily functions, including regulating body temperature, flushing out toxins, and aiding digestion. When following the Galveston Diet, it's important to stay hydrated to support the body's natural detoxification processes and help prevent overeating or mistaking thirst for hunger.

In addition to drinking water, you can also incorporate other hydrating beverages such as herbal tea, coconut water, or infused water with fruits and herbs for added flavor and nutrients. Aim to limit or avoid sugary drinks and alcohol, which can dehydrate the body and negatively impact overall health.

INCORPORATE PHYSICAL ACTIVITY

Adding physical activity to a healthy diet is an effective way to promote weight loss and improve overall health. Regular exercise can increase your metabolism, burn calories, and build muscle mass, which can ultimately lead to weight loss over time. Additionally, physical activity can reduce inflammation, regulate hormone levels, and improve mood and energy levels.

To incorporate exercise into your routine, aim for at least 30 minutes of moderate activity per day. This can include activities like brisk walking, cycling, swimming, or strength training exercises. If you're new to exercise, start slowly and gradually increase the duration and intensity of your workouts. Remember to listen to your body and rest when needed.

Incorporating physical activity into your daily routine can be as simple as taking a walk after dinner or doing a few sets of squats during a commercial break while watching TV. The key is to find activities that you enjoy and can realistically incorporate into your schedule.

Troubleshooting

As with any diet, there may be challenges when following the Galveston Diet. Here are some common challenges and strategies to help overcome them:

1. Cravings: It's common to experience cravings for unhealthy foods when transitioning to a new diet. To overcome this challenge, try incorporating healthy substitutes for your favorite foods. For example, you can swap out chips for roasted chickpeas or fruit for a sweet treat.
2. Eating out: Eating out can be challenging when following a specific diet. To overcome this challenge, research restaurants ahead of time and look for menu options that align with the Galveston Diet principles. You can also consider asking for modifications to menu items to make them more diet-friendly.
3. Time constraints: One of the biggest challenges to healthy eating is time constraints. To overcome this challenge, consider meal prepping on the weekends or during your downtime. This will allow you to have healthy meals and snacks readily available when you're short on time during the week.
4. Lack of variety: Eating the same foods over and over can become boring and lead to burnout. To overcome this challenge, try incorporating new foods and recipes into your diet. Experiment with different herbs and

spices to add variety and flavor to your meals.

5.   Social pressure: Social pressure can make it challenging to stick to a specific diet. To overcome this challenge, be upfront with friends and family about your dietary goals and needs. You can also bring your own healthy dish to social gatherings or suggest restaurants that have menu options that align with the Galveston Diet principles.

6.   Plateaus: It's common to experience weight loss plateaus when following a diet. To overcome this challenge, consider increasing physical activity or making small tweaks to your diet, such as reducing portion sizes or incorporating more protein-rich foods.

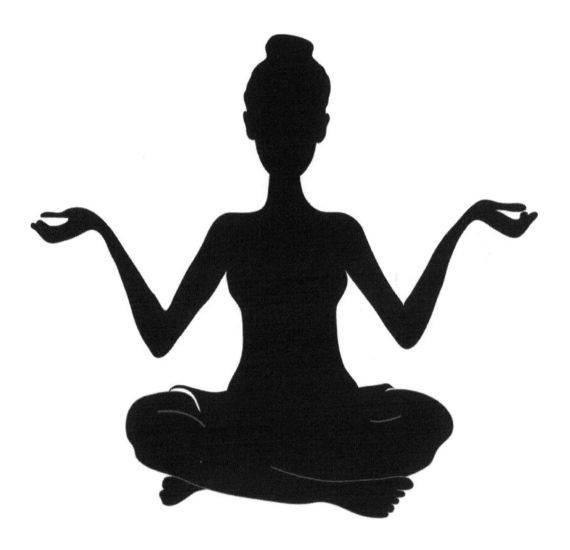

Chapter 3
The Meal Plans and Shopping Lists

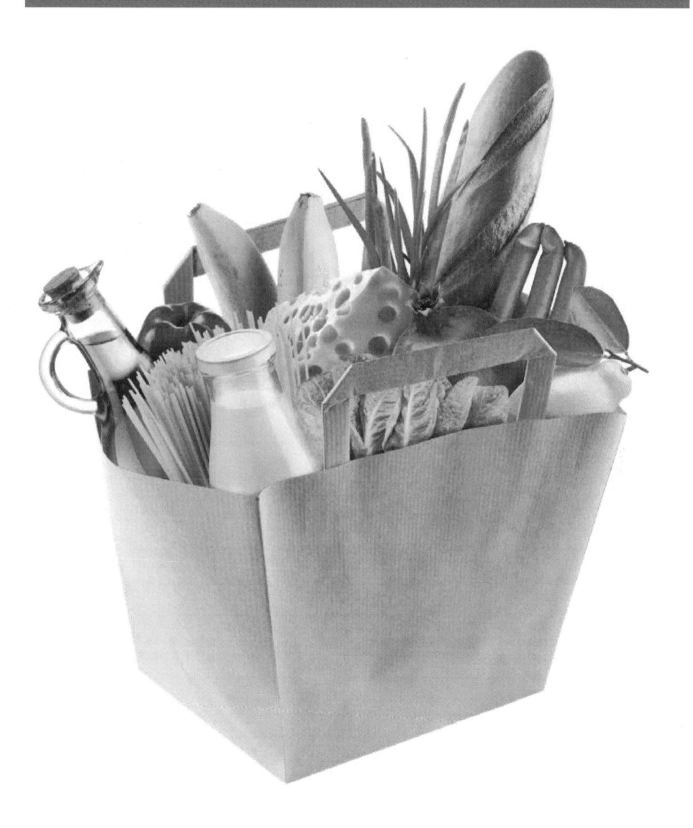

Day 1

Meal 1: Counterfeit Bagels
Snack 1: Jicama Nachos
Meal 2: Chicken Vegetable Soup
Snack 2: Olive Pâté
Macros: Fat: 41.4g, Protein: 38.7g, Net Carbs: 30g, Fiber: 9g

Day 2

Meal 1: Counterfeit Bagels
Snack 1: Jicama Nachos
Meal 2: Chicken Vegetable Soup
Snack 2: Olive Pâté
Macros: Fat: 41.4g, Protein: 38.7g, Net Carbs: 30g, Fiber: 9g

Day 3

Meal 1: Counterfeit Bagels
Snack 1: Jicama Nachos
Meal 2: Chicken Vegetable Soup
Snack 2: Olive Pâté
Macros: Fat: 41.4g, Protein: 38.7g, Net Carbs: 30g, Fiber: 9g

Day 4

Meal 1: Counterfeit Bagels
Snack 1: Jicama Nachos
Meal 2: Chicken Vegetable Soup
Snack 2: Olive Pâté
Macros: Fat: 41.4g, Protein: 38.7g, Net Carbs: 30g, Fiber: 9g

Day 5

Meal 1: Counterfeit Bagels
Snack 1: Jicama Nachos
Meal 2: Chicken Vegetable Soup
Snack 2: Olive Pâté
Macros: Fat: 41.4g, Protein: 38.7g, Net Carbs: 30g, Fiber: 9g

Day 6

Meal 1: Counterfeit Bagels
Snack 1: Jicama Nachos
Meal 2: Chicken Vegetable Soup
Snack 2: Olive Pâté
Macros: Fat: 41.4g, Protein: 38.7g, Net Carbs: 30g, Fiber: 9g

Day 7

Meal 1: Counterfeit Bagels
Snack 1: Haystack Cookies
Meal 2: Chicken Vegetable Soup
Snack 2: Haystack Cookies
Macros: Fat: 41.3g, Protein: 48g, Net Carbs: 7.7g, Fiber: 9.5g

Shopping List for Week 1

Note: Amounts given here indicate the quantities you need for the week's recipes; they are not always indicative of the quantities in which the items are commonly sold.

VEGETABLES:
- ½ medium jicama
- 1 small Roma tomato
- ½ large onion
- 1 bell pepper
- 2 celery stalks
- 2 cups green beans
- 2 cups shredded kale
- 2 garlic cloves
- 1 jalapeño pepper
- 1 (15-ounce) can tomatoes with green chilies
- 1 cup pitted green olives
- 1 cup pitted black olives
- 2 bay leaves

FRUITS:
- 1 lime
- 2 cups (200 g) unsweetened shredded coconut

PROTEINS:
- 1 pound boneless, skinless chicken breasts
- 2½ cups shredded whole milk mozzarella cheese
- 2 ounces full-fat cream cheese

MISCELLANEOUS:
- 1 (32-ounce) carton chicken bone broth
- 1 tablespoon baking powder
- 2 tablespoons Everything but the Bagel seasoning
- 2 tablespoons avocado oil
- 1 tablespoon unsalted butter
- ¼ cup finely diced yellow onion
- 2 thyme sprigs
- 1 teaspoon sea salt
- 2 tablespoons apple cider vinegar
- ½ cup (95 g) erythritol
- ¼ cup (60 ml) full-fat coconut milk
- 3 tablespoons coconut oil, ghee, or cacao butter
- ¼ cup (20 g) cocoa powder
- ⅓ cup (30 g) unflavored MCT oil powder (optional)

Day 1

Meal 1: Radish Hash Browns
Snack 1: Avocado "Fries"
Meal 2: Chicken Creamy Soup
Snack 2: Nutty Chocolate Biscotti
Macros: Fat: 69.5g, Protein: 37g, Net Carbs: 20g, Fiber: 11g

Day 2

Meal 1: Radish Hash Browns
Snack 1: Avocado "Fries"
Meal 2: Chicken Creamy Soup
Snack 2: Nutty Chocolate Biscotti
Macros: Fat: 69.5g, Protein: 37g, Net Carbs: 20g, Fiber: 11g

Day 3

Meal 1: Radish Hash Browns
Snack 1: Avocado "Fries"
Meal 2: Chicken Creamy Soup
Snack 2: Nutty Chocolate Biscotti
Macros: Fat: 69.5g, Protein: 37g, Net Carbs: 20g, Fiber: 11g

Day 4

Meal 1: Radish Hash Browns
Snack 1: Avocado "Fries"
Meal 2: Chicken Creamy Soup
Snack 2: Nutty Chocolate Biscotti
Macros: Fat: 69.5g, Protein: 37g, Net Carbs: 20g, Fiber: 11g

Day 5

Meal 1: Radish Hash Browns
Snack 1: Avocado "Fries"
Meal 2: Choco-Berry Smoothie
Snack 2: Nutty Chocolate Biscotti
Macros: Fat: 69.5g, Protein: 37g, Net Carbs: 20g, Fiber: 11g

Day 6

Meal 1: Radish Hash Browns
Snack 1: Avocado "Fries"
Meal 2: Choco-Berry Smoothie
Snack 2: Nutty Chocolate Biscotti
Macros: Fat: 69.5g, Protein: 37g, Net Carbs: 20g, Fiber: 11g

Day 7

Meal 1: Radish Hash Browns
Snack 1: Nutty Chocolate Biscotti
Meal 2: Choco-Berry Smoothie
Snack 2: Nutty Chocolate Biscotti
Macros: Fat: 30g, Protein: 7g, Net Carbs: 2g, Fiber: 7g

Shopping List for Week 2

VEGETABLES:
- 2 pounds radishes
- 4 tablespoons olive oil
- 1 large egg
- 1/8 teaspoon salt
- 1/8 teaspoon black pepper
- 2 jalapeño peppers
- 2 garlic cloves
- 1 large onion
- 1 bell pepper
- 2 celery stalks
- 2 cups green beans
- 2 cups shredded kale
- 1 (15-ounce) can tomatoes with green chilies
- 1 cup pitted green olives
- 1 cup pitted black olives
- 2 bay leaves

FRUITS:
- Zest of 1 lemon and 1 orange
- 2 cups blackberries
- 1 cup unsweetened shredded coconut
- 1 lime

PROTEINS:
- 2 pounds boneless, skinless chicken breasts
- 1 (32-ounce) carton chicken bone broth

NUTS:
- 1/2 cup pecans or walnuts
- 1 cup almond flour
- 1/2 cup sunflower seeds

MISCELLANEOUS:
- 1 tablespoon ground flaxseed
- 3 tablespoons stevia powder extract
- 2 tablespoons flaxseed meal (ground flax seeds)
- 2 tablespoons finely chopped/shaved bakers' chocolate (100 percent cocoa, no sugar)
- 1 teaspoon pure almond extract
- 1 teaspoon sea salt
- 1/4 teaspoon cayenne pepper
- 1 teaspoon ground paprika
- 1/4 cup monk fruit sweetener
- 1/2 cup shredded whole milk mozzarella cheese
- 2 tbsp poppy seeds
- 2 tbsp pure maple syrup
- 2 tbsp cocoa powder
- 1/3 cup buffalo sauce
- 4 tbsp chopped cilantro

Day 1

Meal 1: Tandoori Chicken Meatballs
Snack 1: Finger Tacos
Meal 2: Cheesy Beef Stroganoff Casserole
Snack 2: Strawberry Shortcake Coconut Ice
Macros: Fat: 88g, Protein: 55g, Net Carbs: 31.5g, Fiber: 15g

Day 2

Meal 1: Tandoori Chicken Meatballs
Snack 1: Finger Tacos
Meal 2: Cheesy Beef Stroganoff Casserole
Snack 2: Strawberry Shortcake Coconut Ice
Macros: Fat: 88g, Protein: 55g, Net Carbs: 31.5g, Fiber: 15g

Day 3

Meal 1: Tandoori Chicken Meatballs
Snack 1: Finger Tacos
Meal 2: Cheesy Beef Stroganoff Casserole
Snack 2: Strawberry Shortcake Coconut Ice
Macros: Fat: 88g, Protein: 55g, Net Carbs: 31.5g, Fiber: 15g

Day 4

Meal 1: Tandoori Chicken Meatballs
Snack 1: Finger Tacos
Meal 2: Cheesy Beef Stroganoff Casserole
Snack 2: Strawberry Shortcake Coconut Ice
Macros: Fat: 88g, Protein: 55g, Net Carbs: 31.5g, Fiber: 15g

Day 5

Meal 1: Tandoori Chicken Meatballs
Snack 1: Oregano Chickpeas
Meal 2: Cheesy Beef Stroganoff Casserole
Snack 2: Oregano Chickpeas
Macros: Fat: 74g, Protein: 60g, Net Carbs: 58.5g, Fiber: 12g

Day 6

Meal 1: Tandoori Chicken Meatballs
Snack 1: Oregano Chickpeas
Meal 2: Cheesy Beef Stroganoff Casserole
Snack 2: Oregano Chickpeas
Macros: Fat: 74g, Protein: 60g, Net Carbs: 58.5g, Fiber: 12g

Day 7

Meal 1: Tandoori Chicken Meatballs
Snack 1: Oregano Chickpeas
Meal 2: Cheesy Beef Stroganoff Casserole
Snack 2: Oregano Chickpeas
Macros: Fat: 74g, Protein: 60g, Net Carbs: 58.5g, Fiber: 12g

Shopping List for Week 3

VEGETABLES:
- 5 tomatoes
- 2 large onions
- 2 tablespoons minced red onions
- 1 head cauliflower
- 1/2 cup kale chiffonade
- 1/2 cup cabbage chiffonade
- 10 fresh mint leaves chiffonade
- 1 teaspoon minced garlic
- 1 teaspoon paprika
- 1/2 teaspoon cayenne pepper
- 1 teaspoon peeled and minced fresh ginger

FRUITS:
- 2 avocados
- 1 lime
- 2 teaspoons lemon juice
- 9 hulled strawberries

PROTEINS:
- 1 pound ground chicken
- 2 pounds stew beef
- 1 large egg, beaten

NUTS:
- 1/2 cup superfine blanched almond flour

MISCELLANEOUS:
- 2 tablespoons full-fat Greek yogurt
- 1 teaspoon kosher salt
- 1/2 teaspoon garam masala
- 1/2 teaspoon ground cumin
- 1/2 teaspoon turmeric powder
- 2 tablespoons avocado oil or other light-tasting oil, for the pan
- 1 tsp extra-virgin olive oil
- 1/2 cup vegetable broth
- 2 tsp dried oregano
- Sea salt and pepper to taste
- 3 tablespoons butter, divided
- 1 tablespoon Worcestershire sauce
- 3/4 cup full-fat sour cream
- 1/4 teaspoon xanthan gum
- 1/2 teaspoon fresh thyme leaves
- 1 batch Cheesy Cauliflower Puree
- 2 tablespoons chopped fresh parsley, for garnish (optional)
- 1 tablespoon tamari
- 1 teaspoon sesame oil
- 1 teaspoon ginger powder
- 1 teaspoon togarashi (optional)
- 1 (0.18-ounce) package nori squares or seaweed snack sheets
- 1 tablespoon apple cider vinegar
- 2 drops liquid stevia, or 2 teaspoons erythritol
- 3 cups (420 g) ice cubes
- 2 (14.5-oz) cans chickpeas

The Conventional Menus: Week 4

Day 1

Meal 1:
Snack 1:
Meal 2:
Snack 2:
Macros: Fat:, Protein:, Net Carbs:, Fiber:

Day 2

Meal 1:
Snack 1:
Meal 2:
Snack 2:
Macros: Fat:, Protein:, Net Carbs:, Fiber:

Day 3

Meal 1:
Snack 1:
Meal 2:
Snack 2:
Macros: Fat:, Protein:, Net Carbs:, Fiber:

Day 4

Meal 1:
Snack 1:
Meal 2:
Snack 2:
Macros: Fat:, Protein:, Net Carbs:, Fiber:

Day 5

Meal 1:
Snack 1:
Meal 2:
Snack 2:
Macros: Fat:, Protein:, Net Carbs:, Fiber:

Day 6

Meal 1:
Snack 1:
Meal 2:
Snack 2:
Macros: Fat:, Protein:, Net Carbs:, Fiber:

Day 7

Meal 1:
Snack 1:
Meal 2:
Snack 2:
Macros: Fat:, Protein:, Net Carbs:, Fiber:

Shopping List for Week 4

Vegetables
Fruits
Proteins
Nuts
Miscellaneous

The Vegetarian Menus: Week 1

Day 1

Meal 1: Celery & Sweet Potato Soup
Snack 1: The Best Keto Fat Bread
Meal 2: Cucumber & Pear Rice Salad
Snack 2: Pistachios & Chocolate Popsicles
Macros: Fat: 24g, Protein: 8g, Net Carbs: 90g, Fiber: 18g

Day 2

Meal 1: Celery & Sweet Potato Soup
Snack 1: The Best Keto Fat Bread
Meal 2: Cucumber & Pear Rice Salad
Snack 2: Pistachios & Chocolate Popsicles
Macros: Fat: 24g, Protein: 8g, Net Carbs: 90g, Fiber: 18g

Day 3

Meal 1: Celery & Sweet Potato Soup
Snack 1: The Best Keto Fat Bread
Meal 2: Cucumber & Pear Rice Salad
Snack 2: Pistachios & Chocolate Popsicles
Macros: Fat: 24g, Protein: 8g, Net Carbs: 90g, Fiber: 18g

Day 4

Meal 1: Celery & Sweet Potato Soup
Snack 1: The Best Keto Fat Bread
Meal 2: Cucumber & Pear Rice Salad
Snack 2: Pistachios & Chocolate Popsicles
Macros: Fat: 24g, Protein: 8g, Net Carbs: 90g, Fiber: 18g

Day 5

Meal 1: Celery & Sweet Potato Soup
Snack 1: The Best Keto Fat Bread
Meal 2: Thai Green Bean & Mango Salad
Snack 2: Paprika Hummus with Mushrooms
Macros: Fat: 25g, Protein: 18g, Net Carbs: 121g, Fiber: 19.4g

Day 6

Meal 1: Celery & Sweet Potato Soup
Snack 1: The Best Keto Fat Bread
Meal 2: Thai Green Bean & Mango Salad
Snack 2: Paprika Hummus with Mushrooms
Macros: Fat: 25g, Protein: 18g, Net Carbs: 121g, Fiber: 19.4g

Day 7

Meal 1: Thai Green Bean & Mango Salad
Snack 1: The Best Keto Fat Bread
Meal 2: Thai Green Bean & Mango Salad
Snack 2: Paprika Hummus with Mushrooms
Macros: Fat:21g, Protein:22g, Net Carbs:144g,
Fiber:20.8g

Shopping List for Vegetarian Week 1

VEGETABLES:
- 1 onion
- 1 carrot
- 1 celery stalk
- 2 garlic cloves
- 1 golden beet
- 1 red bell pepper
- green beans
- 1 cucumber
- mushrooms

FRUITS:
- 1 mango
- 12 cherry tomatoes
- 1 pear
- 1 tbsp lemon juice
- ½ cup lime juice
- ¼ cup orange juice

PROTEINS:
- 5 eggs
- 1 (15-oz) can chickpeas

NUTS:
- 1 cup macadamia nuts
- ½ cup chopped almonds
- 2 tbsp pistachios

MISCELLANEOUS:
- 6 cups vegetable broth
- 1 cup brown rice
- 1 tsp dried thyme
- 1-2 tbsp everything bagel seasoning
- sea salt
- pepper
- 2 oz dark chocolate
- 1 tbsp cocoa powder
- 3 tbsp pure date syrup
- 1 tsp vanilla extract
- ¼ cup raisins
- ¼ cup olive oil
- 3 tbsp extra-virgin olive oil
- ¼ cup tahini
- ½ tsp ground cumin
- ¼ tsp paprika
- sugar-free soy sauce
- raw honey

The Vegetarian Menus: Week 2

Day 1

Meal 1: Buffalo Chili
Snack 1: Pressure Cooked Cherry Pie
Meal 2: Caprese Salad
Snack 2: Smoky "Hummus" And Veggies
Macros: Fat: 38.2g, Protein: 24.9g, Net Carbs: 27.8g,
Fiber: 9.5g

Day 2

Meal 1: Buffalo Chili
Snack 1: : Pressure Cooked Cherry Pie
Meal 2: Caprese Salad
Snack 2: Smoky "Hummus" And Veggies
Macros: Fat: 38.2g, Protein: 24.9g, Net Carbs: 27.8g,
Fiber: 9.5g

Day 3

Meal 1: Buffalo Chili
Snack 1: : Pressure Cooked Cherry Pie
Meal 2: Caprese Salad
Snack 2: Smoky "Hummus" And Veggies
Macros: Fat: 38.2g, Protein: 24.9g, Net Carbs: 27.8g,
Fiber: 9.5g

Day 4

Meal 1: Buffalo Chili
Snack 1: : Pressure Cooked Cherry Pie
Meal 2: Caprese Salad
Snack 2: Smoky "Hummus" And Veggies
Macros: Fat: 38.2g, Protein: 24.9g, Net Carbs: 27.8g,
Fiber: 9.5g

Day 5

Meal 1: Buffalo Chili
Snack 1: : Pressure Cooked Cherry Pie
Meal 2: Caprese Salad
Snack 2: Smoky "Hummus" And Veggies
Macros: Fat: 38.2g, Protein: 24.9g, Net Carbs: 27.8g,
Fiber: 9.5g

Day 6

Meal 1: Buffalo Chili
Snack 1: : Pressure Cooked Cherry Pie
Meal 2: Caprese Salad
Snack 2: Smoky "Hummus" And Veggies
Macros: Fat: 38.2g, Protein: 24.9g, Net Carbs: 27.8g,
Fiber: 9.5g

Day 7

Meal 1: Buffalo Chili
Snack 1: Ranch Kale Chips
Meal 2: Caprese Salad
Snack 2: Ranch Kale Chips
Macros: Fat: 19.9g, Protein: 21.9g, Net Carbs: 20.8g,
Fiber: 7.5g

Shopping List for Vegetarian Week 2

VEGETABLES:
- 1 large poblano pepper
- 1/2 large onion
- 3 garlic cloves
- 4 cups kale
- 1 cauliflower head
- Fresh parsley
- 4 tomatoes
- Celery pieces
- Cucumbers

FRUITS:
- 4 cups cherries

PROTEINS:
- 2 pounds ground bison meat
- Fresh mozzarella cheese

NUTS:
- Pine nuts

MISCELLANEOUS:
- 1 tablespoon coconut oil
- 1 (15-ounce) can roasted tomatoes
- 1 (15-ounce) can tomato sauce (no sugar added)
- 1 cup beef broth
- 1 tsp Ranch seasoning mix
- Balsamic vinegar
- Extra virgin olive oil
- Cold-pressed olive oil
- Tahini
- Quick tapioca
- Brown sugar
- Sea salt
- Black pepper
- Chili powder
- Ground cumin
- Almond extract
- Vanilla extract
- Smoked paprika
- Flax crackers
- Avocado (optional)
- Grass-fed shredded cheese (optional)
- Sour cream (optional)

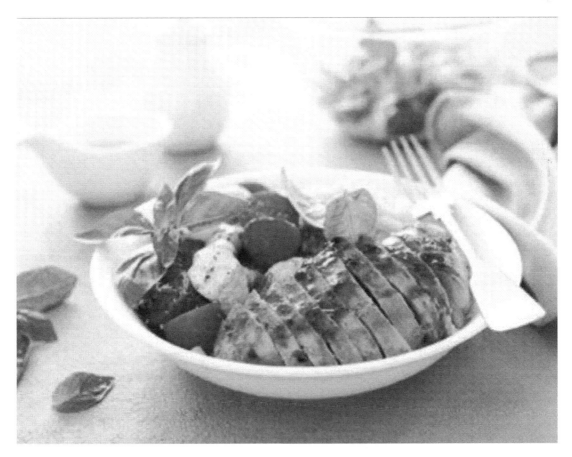

Chapter 4
Snacks & Sides

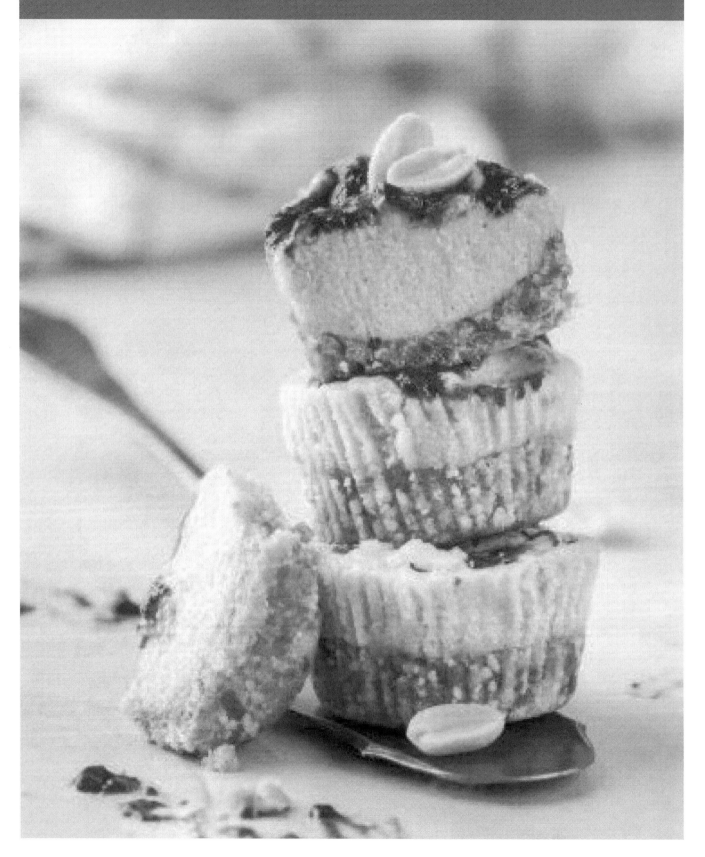

Broccoli Stir-Fry with Sesame Seeds
Prep time: 5 minutes | Cook time: 15 minutes | Serves 4

- 1 tbsp cilantro, chopped
- 2 tbsp canola oil
- 1 tsp sesame oil
- 4 cups broccoli florets
- 1 tbsp grated fresh ginger
- ¼ tsp sea salt
- 2 garlic cloves, minced
- 2 tbsp toasted sesame seeds

1. Warm the canola oil in a skillet over medium heat and place in the broccoli, ginger, garlic, and salt.
2. Cook for 5-7 minutes until the broccoli gets brown.
3. Add in garlic and cook for another 30 seconds.
4. Turn the heat off and mix in sesame seeds.
5. Top with cilantro and serve immediately.

PER SERVING

Cal 140| Fat 12g| Carbs 10g| Protein 3g

Garlicky Roasted Vegetables
Prep time: 5 minutes | Cook time:25 minutes | Serves 4

- 1 red bell pepper, chopped
- 1 red onion, chopped
- 2 zucchini, chopped
- 1 yellow bell pepper, chopped
- 1 sweet potato, chopped
- 4 garlic cloves, minced
- ¼ cup extra-virgin olive oil
- Sea salt to taste

1. Preheat the oven to 450°F.
2. Line a baking sheet with foil.
3. Combine the bell pepper, onion, zucchini, sweet potato, olive oil, salt, and garlic in a bowl.
4. Place it on the sheet and bake for 25 minutes, turning once.
5. Serve warm.

PER SERVING

Cal 185| Fat 13g| Carbs 16g| Protein 2g

Avocado "Fries"
Prep time: 10 minutes | Cook time: 15 minutes | Serves 6

- 1 or 2 medium semi-firm avocado(s), peeled, pitted, and cut lengthwise into 1-inch-thick sticks
- 1 cup almond flour
- 1 tablespoon ground flaxseed
- 1 teaspoon ground paprika
- ¼ teaspoon cayenne pepper
- 1 cup unsweetened hemp milk
- 1 teaspoon sea salt

1. Preheat the oven to 420°F. Line a baking sheet with parchment paper. If you don't have parchment paper, use aluminum foil or a greased pan.
2. In a mixing bowl, whisk together the almond flour, flaxseed, paprika, and cayenne.
3. Pour the hemp milk into a separate bowl and set aside.
4. Dip the avocado sticks in the hemp milk, then immediately roll them in the dry mixture until well coated. Place the coated avocado sticks on the prepared baking sheet.
5. Bake for 7 minutes on one side, then flip the fries and bake for another 5 minutes until golden brown and crisp.
6. Remove the fries from the oven and sprinkle with the salt.

PER SERVING

Calories: 170 | Total Fat: 16g | Carbohydrates: 5g | Fiber: 3g | Net Carbs: 2g | Protein: 7g

Jicama Nachos
Prep time: 10 minutes | Cook time: 5 minutes | Serves 6

- 1 lime, halved
- ½ medium jicama, peeled and thinly sliced
- 1 cup "Nacho Cheese" Sauce
- 1 small Roma tomato, finely diced
- ¼ cup finely diced yellow onion
- 1 jalapeño pepper, seeded and finely diced
- ¼ cup sliced olives
- 2 tablespoons coarsely chopped fresh cilantro

1. In a medium bowl, squeeze the lime halves directly over the jicama and set the jicama aside.
2. In a small saucepan, heat the "nacho cheese" until it is warm and a little steam is rising from the surface. If the cheese becomes too thick, stir in a little water to thin it out.
3. Arrange the jicama "nacho chips" on a plate and pour the "nacho cheese" on top.
4. Top with the tomato, onion, and jalapeño.
5. Finish by sprinkling the nachos with the olives and cilantro.

PER SERVING

Calories: 79 | Total Fat: 4g | Carbohydrates: 11g | Fiber: 5gm | Net Carbs: 6g | Protein: 3g

Smoky "Hummus" And Veggies

Prep time: 15 minutes | Cook time: 20 minutes | Serves 6

- Nonstick coconut oil cooking spray
- 1 cauliflower head, cut into florets
- ¼ cup tahini
- ¼ cup cold-pressed olive oil, plus extra for drizzling
- Juice of 1 lemon
- 1 tablespoon ground paprika
- 1 teaspoon sea salt
- ¼ cup chopped fresh parsley, for garnish
- 2 tablespoons pine nuts (optional)
- Flax crackers, for serving
- Sliced cucumbers, for serving
- Celery pieces, for serving

1. Preheat the oven to 400°F and grease a baking sheet with cooking spray.
2. Spread the cauliflower florets out on the prepared baking sheet and bake for 20 minutes.
3. Remove the cauliflower from the oven and allow it to cool for 10 minutes.
4. In a food processor or high-powered blender, combine the cauliflower with the tahini, olive oil, lemon juice, paprika, and salt. Blend on high until a fluffy, creamy texture is achieved. If the mixture seems too thick, slowly add a few tablespoons of water until smooth.
5. Scoop the "hummus" into an airtight container and chill in the refrigerator for about 20 minutes.
6. Transfer the "hummus" to a serving bowl and drizzle with olive oil. Garnish with the parsley and pine nuts (if using).
7. Serve with your favorite flax crackers and sliced cucumbers and celery.

PER SERVING

Calories: 169 | Total Fat: 15g | Carbohydrates: 9g | Fiber: 4g | Net Carbs: 5g | Protein: 4g

Finger Tacos

Prep time: 15 minutes | Cook time: 15 minutes | Serves 4

- 2 avocados, peeled and pitted
- 1 lime
- 1 tablespoon tamari
- 1 teaspoon sesame oil
- 1 teaspoon ginger powder
- 1 teaspoon togarashi (optional)
- ½ cup kale chiffonade
- ½ cup cabbage chiffonade
- 10 fresh mint leaves chiffonade
- ⅓ cup cauliflower rice
- 1 (0.18-ounce) package nori squares or seaweed snack sheets

1. Put the avocados into a large mixing bowl, and squeeze the lime over them.
2. Roughly mash the avocados with a fork, leaving the mixture fairly chunky.
3. Gently stir in the tamari, sesame oil, ginger powder, and togarashi (if using).
4. Gently fold in the kale, cabbage, mint, and cauliflower rice.
5. Arrange some nori squares on a plate.
6. Use a nori or seaweed sheet to pick up a portion of the avocado mixture and pop it into your mouth.

PER SERVING

Calories: 180 | Total Fat: 15g | Carbohydrates: 13g | Fiber: 8g | Net Carbs: 5g | Protein: 4g

Pepita Cheese Tomato Chips

Prep time: 5 minutes | Cook time:10 minutes | Serves 6

- 5 tomatoes, sliced
- ¼ cup extra-virgin olive oil
- ½ cup pepitas seeds
- 1 tbsp nutritional yeast
- Sea salt and pepper to taste
- 1 tsp garlic puree

1. Preheat your oven to 400°F.
2. Over the sliced tomatoes, drizzle olive oil.
3. In a food processor, add pepitas seeds, nutritional yeast, garlic, salt, and pepper and pulse until the desired consistency is attained.
4. Toss in tomato slices to coat.
5. Set the tomato slices on a baking pan and bake for 10 minutes.
6. Serve and enjoy!

PER SERVING

Cal 150| Fat 14g| Carbs 6g| Protein 4g| Fiber: 4g

Oregano Chickpeas

Prep time: 5 minutes | Cook time:5 minutes | Serves 6

- 1 tsp extra-virgin olive oil
- 1 onion, sliced
- 2 (14.5-oz) cans chickpeas
- ½ cup vegetable broth
- 2 tsp dried oregano
- Sea salt and pepper to taste

1. Heat the oil in a skillet over medium heat.
2. Cook the onion for 3 minutes.
3. Stir in chickpeas, broth, oregano, salt, and pepper.
4. Bring to a boil and simmer for 10 minutes.
5. Serve.

PER SERVING

Cal 130| Fat 3g| Carbs 20g| Protein 6g| Fiber: 3g

Paprika Hummus with Mushrooms

Prep time: 5 minutes | Cook time:10 minutes | Serves 4

- 1 (15-oz) can chickpeas
- Juice of 1 lemon
- ¼ cup tahini
- 3 tbsp extra-virgin olive oil
- ½ tsp ground cumin
- 1 tbsp water
- ¼ tsp paprika
- 1 lb sautéed mushrooms

1. In a blender, put the chickpeas, lemon juice, tahini, 2 tbsp of olive oil, cumin, and water.
2. Pulse for 30 seconds until ingredients are evenly mixed.
3. Sprinkle with the remaining olive oil and paprika.
4. Serve with mushrooms.

PER SERVING

Cal 605| Fat 21g| Carbs 104g| Protein 18g| Fiber: 6g

Spicy Nut Burgers

Prep time: 5 minutes | Cook time:15 minutes | Serves 4

- ¾ cup chopped walnuts
- ¾ cup chopped cashews
- 1 medium carrot, grated
- 1 small onion, chopped
- 1 garlic clove, minced
- 1 serrano pepper, minced
- ¾ cup old-fashioned oats
- ¾ cup breadcrumbs
- 2 tbsp minced cilantro
- ½ tsp ground coriander
- Sea salt and pepper to taste
- 2 tsp fresh lime juice
- 2 tbsp extra-virgin olive oil
- 4 sandwich rolls
- Lettuce leaves for garnish

1. Pulse walnuts, cashews, carrot, onion, garlic, serrano pepper, oats, breadcrumbs, cilantro, coriander, lime juice, salt, and pepper in a food processor until well mixed.
2. Remove and form into 4 burgers.
3. Warm the olive oil in a skillet over medium heat.
4. Cook the burgers for 5 minutes per side until golden brown.
5. Serve in sandwich rolls with lettuce and a dressing of your choice.

PER SERVING

Cal 570| Fat 38g| Carbs 54g| Protein 16g

Beet & Carrot Stir-Fry

Prep time: 5 minutes | Cook time: 15 minutes | Serves 4

- 2 peeled beets, cut into wedges
- 3 carrots, cut crosswise
- 2 tbsp extra-virgin olive oil
- 1 red onion, cut into wedges
- ½ tsp dried oregano
- Sea salt to taste

1. Steam the beets and carrots in a microwave bowl until softened, 6 minutes.
2. Warm the olive oil in a large skillet and sauté the onion until softened, 3 minutes.
3. Stir in the carrots, beets, oregano, and salt.
4. Mix well and cook for 5 minutes.
5. Serve warm.

PER SERVING

Cal 105| Fat 7g| Carbs 10g| Protein 1g

Garbanzo Quesadillas with Salsa

Prep time: 5 minutes | Cook time:10 minutes | Serves 4

- 1 (15.5-oz) can garbanzo beans, mashed
- 2 tbsp extra-virgin olive oil
- 1 tsp chili powder
- 8 whole-wheat flour tortillas
- 1 cup tomato salsa
- ½ cup minced red onion

1. Warm the olive oil in a pot over medium heat.
2. Place in mashed garbanzo and chili powder, cook for 5 minutes, stirring often.
3. Set aside.
4. Heat a pan over medium heat.
5. Put one tortilla in the pan and top with ¼ each of the garbanzo spread, tomato salsa, and onion.
6. Cover with other tortillas and cook for 2 minutes, flip the quesadilla and cook for another 2 minutes until crispy.
7. Repeat the process with the remaining tortillas.
8. Slice and serve.

PER SERVING

Cal 345| Fat 15g| Carbs 44g| Protein 10g

Olive Pâté

Prep time: 10 minutes | Cook time: 15 minutes | Serves 6

- 1 cup pitted green olives
- 1 cup pitted black olives
- ¼ cup cold-pressed olive oil
- 1 teaspoon freshly ground black pepper
- 2 thyme sprigs

1. In a food processor, combine all the ingredients and pulse until the mixture is thick and chunky.
2. Transfer the pâté to a small serving bowl and serve with crackers.

PER SERVING

Calories: 171 | Total Fat: 17g | Carbohydrates: 4g | Fiber: <1g | Net Carbs: 4g | Protein: <1g

Ranch Kale Chips

Prep time: 5 minutes | Cook time:20 minutes | Serves 2

- 2 tbsp extra-virgin olive oil
- 4 cups kale, torn
- 1 tsp sea salt
- 1 tsp Ranch seasoning mix

1. Preheat your oven to 350°F.
2. Combine all the ingredients in a large bowl.
3. Stir to mix well.
4. Gently massage the kale leaves in the bowl for 5 minutes or until wilted and bright.
5. Place the kale on a baking sheet.
6. Bake in the oven for 20 minutes or until crispy.
7. Toss the kale halfway through.

PER SERVING

Cal 140| Fat 15g| Carbs 3g| Protein 1g| Fiber: 2g

Ketone Gummies

Prep time: 10 minutes | Cook time:5 minutes |Serves 1

- ½ cup (120 ml) lemon juice
- 8 hulled strawberries (fresh or frozen and defrosted)
- 2 tablespoons unflavored gelatin
- 2 teaspoons exogenous ketones
- Special Equipment (Optional):
- Silicone mold with eight 2-tablespoon or larger cavities

1. Have on hand your favorite silicone mold. I like to use a large silicone ice cube tray and spoon 2 tablespoons of the mixture into each cavity, which makes 8 gummies total. If you do not have a silicone mold, you can use an 8-inch (20-cm) square silicone or metal baking pan; if using a metal pan, line it with parchment paper, draping some over the sides for easy removal.
2. Place the lemon juice, strawberries, and gelatin in a blender or food processor and pulse until smooth. Transfer the mixture to a small saucepan and set over low heat for 5 minutes, or until it becomes very liquid-y and begins to simmer.
3. Remove from the heat and stir in the exogenous ketones.
4. Divide the mixture evenly among 8 cavities of the mold or pour into the baking pan. Transfer to the fridge and allow to set for 30 minutes. If using a baking pan, cut into 8 squares.

PER SERVING

Calories: 19 | Calories From Fat: 1.8 | Total Fat: 0.2 g | Saturated Fat: 0.1 g | Cholesterol: 0 mg | Sodium: 10 mg | Carbs: 1.2 g | Dietary Fiber: 0.3 g | Net Carbs: 0.9 g | Sugars: 0.9 g | Protein: 3.2 g

Strawberry Shortcake Coconut Ice

Prep time: 15 minutes | Cook time:5 minutes |Serves 4

- 9 hulled strawberries (fresh or frozen and defrosted)
- ⅓ cup (85 g) coconut cream
- 1 tablespoon apple cider vinegar
- 2 drops liquid stevia, or 2 teaspoons erythritol
- 3 cups (420 g) ice cubes

1. Place the strawberries, coconut cream, vinegar, and sweetener in a blender or food processor. Blend until smooth.
2. Add the ice and pulse until crushed.
3. Divide among four ¾-cup (180-ml) or larger bowls and serve immediately.

PER SERVING

Calories: 61 | Calories From Fat: 45 | Total Fat: 5 g | Saturated Fat: 4.4 g | Cholesterol: 0 mg | Sodium: 4 mg | Carbs: 3.3 g | Dietary Fiber: 1 g | Net Carbs: 2.3 g | Sugars: 2 g | Protein: 0.7 g

Haystack Cookies

Prep time: 10 minutes | Cook time:5 minutes |Serves 2

- ½ cup (95 g) erythritol
- ¼ cup (60 ml) full-fat coconut milk
- 3 tablespoons coconut oil, ghee, or cacao butter
- ¼ cup (20 g) cocoa powder
- ⅓ cup (30 g) unflavored MCT oil powder (optional)
- 2 cups (200 g) unsweetened shredded coconut

1. Line a rimmed baking sheet or large plate with parchment paper or a silicone baking mat.
2. Place the erythritol, coconut milk, and oil in a large frying pan. Slowly bring to a simmer over medium-low heat, whisking periodically to prevent burning; this should take about 5 minutes.
3. When the mixture reaches a simmer, remove from the heat and stir in the cocoa powder. Once fully combined, stir in the MCT oil powder, if using, and then the shredded coconut.
4. Using a 1-tablespoon measuring spoon, carefully scoop out a portion of the mixture and press it into the spoon. Place the haystack on the lined baking sheet and repeat, making a total of 20 cookies.
5. Refrigerate for 30 to 45 minutes before enjoying.

PER SERVING

Calories: 122 | Calories From Fat: 107 | Total Fat: 11.9 g | Saturated Fat: 9.6 g | Cholesterol: 0 mg | Sodium: 4 mg | Carbs: 4.2 g | Dietary Fiber: 2.5 g | Net Carbs: 1.7 g | Sugars: 1.2 g | Protein: 1.3 g

Grandma'S Meringues

Prep time: 10 minutes | Cook time:1 minutes |Serves 2

- 2 large egg whites, room temperature
- ¼ teaspoon cream of tartar
- Pinch of finely ground sea salt
- ½ cup (80 g) confectioners'-style erythritol
- ½ teaspoon vanilla extract
- For Serving:
- 24 fresh strawberries, sliced
- ¾ cup (190 g) coconut cream
- 12 fresh mint leaves

1. Preheat the oven to 225°F (108°C). Line a rimmed baking sheet with parchment paper or a silicone baking mat.
2. Place the egg whites, cream of tartar, and salt in a very clean large bowl. Make sure that the bowl does not have any oil residue in it. Using a handheld electric mixer or stand mixer, mix on low speed until the mixture becomes foamy.
3. Once foamy, increase the speed to high. Slowly add the erythritol, 1 tablespoon at a time, mixing all the while. Add a tablespoon about every 20 seconds.
4. Keep beating until the mixture is shiny and thick and peaks have formed; it should be nearly doubled in volume. (The peaks won't be as stiff as in a traditional meringue.) Fold in the vanilla.
5. Using a large spoon, dollop the meringue mixture onto the lined baking sheet, making a total of 12 meringues.
6. Bake for 1 hour without opening the oven door. After 1 hour, turn off the oven and keep the meringues in the cooling oven for another hour, then remove.
7. To serve, place 2 meringues on each plate. Top each serving with 4 sliced strawberries, 2 tablespoons of coconut cream, and 2 mint leaves.

PER SERVING

Calories: 100 | Calories From Fat: 68 | Total Fat: 7.6 g | Saturated Fat: 6.6 g | Cholesterol: 0 mg | Sodium: 56 mg | Carbs: 5.8 g | Dietary Fiber: 1.8 g | Net Carbs: 4 g | Sugars: 3.5 g | Protein: 2.3 g

Roman Balsamic Tomato Bruschetta

Prep time: 5 minutes | Cook time:15minutes | Serves 4

- 3 tomatoes, chopped
- ¼ cup chopped basil
- 1 tbsp extra-virgin olive oil
- 1 whole-wheat baguette, sliced
- 1 garlic clove, halved
- 1 tbsp balsamic vinegar

1. Preheat your oven to 420°F.
2. Mix the tomatoes, basil, olive oil, and salt in a bowl.
3. Set aside.
4. Arrange baguette slices on a baking sheet and toast for 6 minutes on both sides until brown.
5. Spread the garlic over the bread and top with the tomato mixture.
6. Serve right away.

PER SERVING

Cal 50| Fat 4g| Carbs 5g| Protein 1g

Classic Guacamole

Prep time: 5 minutes | Cook time:5 minutes | Serves 4

- 2 tbsp extra-virgin olive oil
- 2 ripe avocados, cubed
- 2 tomatoes, diced
- ½ red onion, minced
- 2 tbsp chopped cilantro
- ½ tsp sea salt

1. Put the olive oil, avocados, tomatoes, red onion, cilantro, and sea salt in a medium bowl.
2. Mash them lightly with the back of a fork until a uniform consistency is achieved.

PER SERVING

Cal 215| Fat 20g| Carbs 10g| Protein 3g

French Mushroom Tarts

Prep time: 5 minutes | Cook time:15 minutes | Serves 4

- 12 whole-grain bread slices
- 1 tbsp extra-virgin olive oil + more for brushing
- 2 spring onions, chopped
- 2 garlic cloves, minced
- 12 oz mushrooms, chopped
- ¼ cup chopped cilantro
- 1 tsp dried thyme
- 1 tsp low-sodium soy sauce

1. Preheat your oven to 390°F.
2. Using a small round tin, make circles from the bread slices.
3. Coat the circles with oil and press at the bottom of a muffin tin.
4. Bake for 10 minutes, until toasted.
5. Heat 1 tbsp of oil in a skillet over medium heat.
6. Place in spring onions, garlic, and mushrooms and cook for 5 minutes, until tender.
7. Add in cilantro, thyme, and soy sauce and cook for 2-3 minutes more, until liquid has absorbed.
8. Divide the mixture between the muffin cups and bake for 3-5 minutes.
9. Serve.

PER SERVING

Cal 370| Fat 7g| Carbs 59g| Protein 19g

Chapter 5
Breakfast & Smoothies

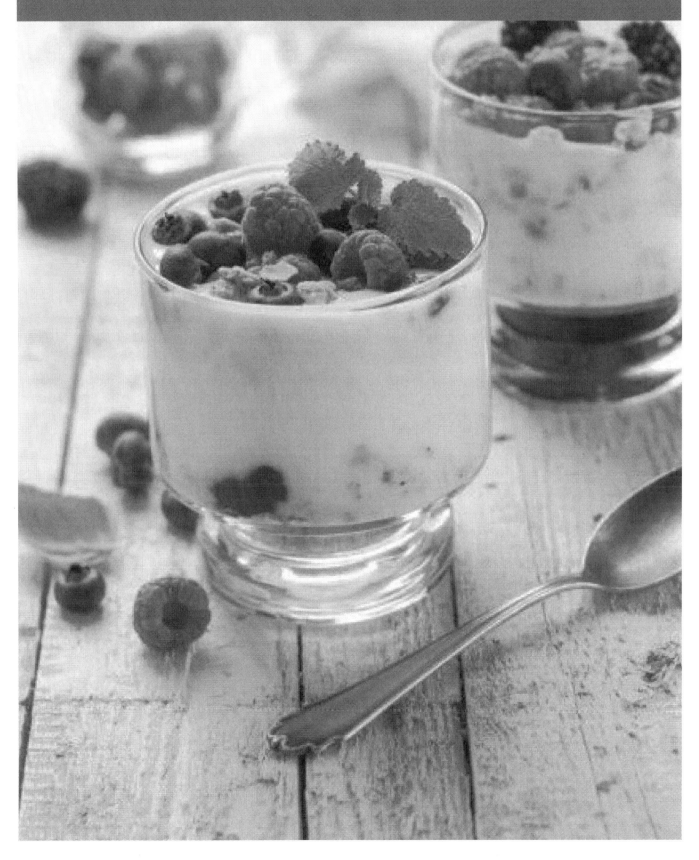

Pear & Kale Smoothie

Prep time: 5 minutes | Cook time:5 minutes | Serves 2

- 3 cups baby kale
- ¼ cup cilantro leaves
- 2 pears, peeled and chopped
- 2 cups sugar-free apple juice
- 1 tbsp grated ginger
- 1 cup crushed ice

1. Place the kale, cilantro, pears, apple juice, ginger, and ice in a food processor and pulse until smooth.
2. Serve.

PER SERVING

Cal 310| Fat 2g| Carbs 78g| Protein 2g

Blueberry Muesli Breakfast

Prep time: 5 minutes | Cook time:5 minutes | Serves 4

- 2 cups spelt flakes
- 2 cups puffed cereal
- ¼ cup sunflower seeds
- ¼ cup almonds
- ¼ cup raisins
- ¼ cup dried cranberries
- ¼ cup chopped dried figs
- ¼ cup shredded coconut
- ¼ cup dark chocolate chips
- 3 tsp ground cinnamon
- ½ cup coconut milk
- ½ cup blueberries

1. In a bowl, combine the spelt flakes, puffed cereal, sunflower seeds, almonds, raisins, cranberries, figs, coconut, chocolate chips, and cinnamon.
2. Toss to mix well.
3. Pour in the coconut milk.
4. Let sit for 1 hour and serve topped with blueberries.

PER SERVING

Cal 333| Fat 15g| Carbs 49g| Protein 6.2g

Chocolate-Mango Quinoa Bowl

Prep time: 5 minutes | Cook time:30 minutes | Serves 2

- 1 cup quinoa
- 1 tsp ground cinnamon
- 1 cup non-dairy milk
- 1 large mango, chopped
- 3 tbsp cocoa powder
- 2 tbsp almond butter
- 1 tbsp hemp seeds
- 1 tbsp walnuts
- ¼ cup raspberries

1. In a pot, combine the quinoa, cinnamon, milk, and 1 cup of water over medium heat.
2. Bring to a boil, low heat, and simmer covered for 25-30 minutes.
3. In a bowl, mash the mango and mix cocoa powder, almond butter, and hemp seeds.
4. In a serving bowl, place cooked quinoa and mango mixture.
5. Top with walnuts and raspberries.
6. Serve.

PER SERVING

Cal 584| Fat 21g| Carbs 83g| Protein 23.4g

Pepper Sausage Fry

Prep time: 5 minutes | Cook time:20 minutes |Serves 4

- ¼ cup (60 ml) avocado oil, or ¼ cup (55 g) coconut oil
- 12 ounces (340 g) smoked sausages, thinly sliced
- 1 small green bell pepper, thinly sliced
- 1 small red bell pepper, thinly sliced
- 1½ teaspoons garlic powder
- 1 teaspoon dried oregano leaves
- 1 teaspoon paprika
- ¼ teaspoon finely ground sea salt
- ¼ teaspoon ground black pepper
- ¼ cup (17 g) chopped fresh parsley

1. Heat the oil in a large frying pan over medium-low heat until it shimmers.
2. When the oil is shimmering, add the rest of the ingredients, except the parsley. Cover and cook for 15 minutes, until the bell peppers are fork-tender.
3. Remove the lid and continue to cook for 5 to 6 minutes, until the liquid evaporates.
4. Remove from the heat, stir in the parsley, and serve.

PER SERVING

Calories: 411 | Calories From Fat: 345 | Total Fat: 38.3 g | Saturated Fat: 9.9 g | Cholesterol: 49 mg | Sodium: 903 mg | Carbs: 6.3 g | Dietary Fiber: 1.5 g | Net Carbs: 4.8 g | Sugars: 1.9 g | Protein: 11.1 g

Lemony Quinoa Muffins

Prep time: 5 minutes | Cook time:20 minutes | Serves 4

- 2 tbsp coconut oil melted
- ¼ cup ground flaxseed
- 2 cups lemon curd
- ½ cup pure date sugar
- 1 tsp apple cider vinegar
- 2 ½ cups whole-wheat flour
- 1 ½ cups cooked quinoa
- 2 tsp baking soda
- A pinch of sea salt
- ½ cup raisins

1. Preheat your oven to 400°F.
2. In a bowl, combine the flaxseed and ½ cup water.
3. Stir in the lemon curd, sugar, coconut oil, and vinegar.
4. Add in flour, quinoa, baking soda, and salt.
5. Put in the raisins, be careful not too fluffy.
6. Divide the batter between greased muffin tin and bake for 20 minutes until golden and set.
7. Allow cooling slightly before removing it from the tin.
8. Serve.

PER SERVING

Cal 719| Fat 11g| Carbs 133g| Protein 19g

Keto Breakfast Pudding

Prep time: 5 minutes | Cook time:5 minutes |Serves 3

- 1½ cups (350 ml) full-fat coconut milk
- 1 cup (110 g) frozen raspberries
- ¼ cup (60 ml) MCT oil or melted coconut oil, or ¼ cup (40 g) unflavored MCT oil powder
- ¼ cup (40 g) collagen peptides or protein powder
- 2 tablespoons chia seeds
- 1 tablespoon apple cider vinegar
- 1 teaspoon vanilla extract
- 1 tablespoon erythritol, or 4 drops liquid stevia
- Toppings (Optional):
- Unsweetened shredded coconut
- Hulled hemp seeds
- Fresh berries of choice

1. Place all the pudding ingredients in a blender or food processor and blend until smooth.
2. Serve in bowls with your favorite toppings, if desired.

PER SERVING

Calories: 403 | Calories From Fat: 308 | Total Fat: 34.2 g | Saturated Fat: 30.8 g | Cholesterol: 0 mg | Sodium: 99 mg | Carbs: 8.8 g | Dietary Fiber: 3.1 g | Net Carbs: 5.7 g | Sugars: 3.4 g | Protein: 15.2 g

Carrot-Strawberry Smoothie

Prep time: 5 minutes | Cook time:5minutes | Serves 2

- 1 cup diced carrots
- 1 cup strawberries
- 1 apple, chopped
- 2 tbsp maple syrup
- 2 cups almond milk

1. Place in a food processor all the ingredients.
2. Blitz until smooth.
3. Pour in glasses and serve.

PER SERVING

Cal 708| Fat 58g| Carbs 53.4g| Protein 7g

Mug Biscuit

Prep time: 1 minutes | Cook time:2 minutes |Serves 1

- ¼ cup (28 g) blanched almond flour
- 1 tablespoon coconut flour
- ½ teaspoon baking powder
- ¼ teaspoon finely ground sea salt
- 1 large egg
- 1 tablespoon softened coconut oil or ghee, plus more for serving if desired
- 1 teaspoon apple cider vinegar

1. Place all the ingredients in a microwave-safe mug with a base at least 2 inches (5 cm) in diameter. Mix until fully incorporated, then flatten with the back of a spoon.
2. Place the mug in the microwave and cook on high for 1 minute 30 seconds.
3. Remove the mug from the microwave and insert a toothpick. It should come out clean. If batter is clinging to the toothpick, microwave the biscuit for an additional 15 to 30 seconds.
4. Flip the mug over a clean plate and shake it a bit until the biscuit releases from the mug. If desired, slather the biscuit with the fat of your choice while still warm.

PER SERVING

Calories: 399 | Calories From Fat: 302 | Total Fat: 33.5 g | Saturated Fat: 14.6 g | Cholesterol: 164 mg | Sodium: 535 mg | Carbs: 10.6 g | Dietary Fiber: 5.5 g | Net Carbs: 5.1 g | Sugars: 1.9 g | Protein: 13.8 g

Coconut Flaxseed Waffles

Prep time: 15 minutes | Cook time:5 minutes |Serves 4

- Nonstick cooking spray
- 5 eggs
- ½ cup water
- ⅓ cup coconut oil, melted
- 2 cups ground flaxseed
- 1 tablespoon baking powder
- 1 teaspoon salt
- 2 tablespoons unsweetened coconut flakes
- 5 to 6 drops liquid stevia
- 4 tablespoons grass-fed butter

1. Spray a waffle iron with cooking spray and heat it to a medium-high temperature. Allow ample time for it to get up to temperature.
2. Combine the eggs, water, and coconut oil in a blender. Blend on high speed for 30 to 40 seconds.
3. In a medium bowl, mix together the flaxseed, baking powder, and salt until combined.
4. Pour the blender mixture into the flaxseed blend and stir. Allow to sit for 4 to 5 minutes to thicken.
5. Add the coconut flakes and stevia, and then mix well to combine.
6. Pour ¼ cup of batter for each waffle onto the waffle iron and allow to cook thoroughly. Repeat until all the batter has been used.
7. Top each waffle with 1 tablespoon of grass-fed butter.

PER SERVING

Calories: 498 | Fat: 46g | Protein: 12g | Total Carbs: 9g | Net Carbs: 2g | Fiber: 7g | Sugar: 0g | Sodium: 162mg | Macros: Fat: 83% | Protein: 10% | Carbs: 7%

Dlk Bulletproof Coffee

Prep time: 2 minutes | Cook time: 10 minutes | Serves 1

- 1 tablespoon MCT oil
- 8 ounces hot brewed coffee

1. Add MCT oil to coffee and blend using a hand immersion blender until froth whips up. This will help prevent the dreaded MCT oil "."
2. Serve.

PER SERVING

Calories: 132 | Fat: 14g | Protein: 0g | Sodium: 4mg| Fiber: 0g |Carbohydrates: 0g | Net Carbs: 0g | Sugar: 0g

Indian Masala Omelet

Prep time: 8 minutes | Cook time:25 minutes |Serves 2

- 3 tablespoons avocado oil, coconut oil, or ghee
- ¼ cup (20 g) sliced green onions
- 1 clove garlic, minced
- 1 small tomato, diced
- 1 green chili pepper, seeded and finely diced
- 1½ teaspoons curry powder
- ½ teaspoon garam masala
- 6 large eggs, beaten
- ¼ cup (15 g) chopped fresh cilantro leaves and stems

1. Heat the oil in a large frying pan over medium heat until it shimmers. When the oil is shimmering, add the green onions, garlic, tomato, and chili pepper. Cook for 10 minutes, or until the liquid from the tomatoes has evaporated.
2. Reduce the heat to low and sprinkle the tomato mixture with the curry powder and garam masala. Stir to incorporate, then drizzle the beaten eggs over the top.
3. Cover and cook for 5 minutes, or until the edges are cooked through.
4. Sprinkle with the cilantro, fold one side over the other, cover, and cook for another 10 minutes.
5. Remove from the heat, cut in half, and serve.

PER SERVING

Calories: 438 | Calories From Fat: 327 | Total Fat: 36.3 g | Saturated Fat: 7.1 g | Cholesterol: 558 mg | Sodium: 279 mg | Carbs: 7.7 g | Dietary Fiber: 1.9 g | Net Carbs: 5.8 g | Sugars: 4.2 g | Protein: 20.2 g

Morning Pecan & Pear Farro
Prep time: 5 minutes | Cook time:15 minutes | Serves 4

- 1 cup farro
- 1 tbsp peanut butter
- 2 pears, peeled and chopped
- ¼ cup chopped pecans

1. Bring salted water to a boil in a pot over high heat.
2. Stir in farro.
3. Lower the heat, cover, and simmer for 15 minutes until the farro is tender and the liquid has absorbed.
4. Turn the heat off and add in the peanut butter, pears, and pecans.
5. Cover and rest for 12-15 minutes.
6. Serve.

PER SERVING

Cal 387| Fat 28g| Carbs 32g| Protein 8.6g

Creamy Sesame Bread
Prep time: 5 minutes | Cook time:35 minutes | Serves 6

- 4 eggs
- 2/3 cup Greek yogurt
- 4 tbsp olive oil
- 1 cup coconut flour
- 2 tbsp psyllium husk powder
- 1 tsp sea salt
- 1 tsp baking powder
- 1 tbsp sesame seeds

1. Preheat your oven to 400°F.
2. Beat the eggs with yogurt and olive oil until well mixed.
3. Whisk in the coconut flour, psyllium husk powder, salt, and baking powder until adequately blended.
4. Grease a 9 x 5 inches baking tray with cooking spray, and spread the dough in the tray.
5. Allow the mixture to stand for 5 minutes and then brush with some sesame oil.
6. Sprinkle with the sesame seeds and bake the dough for 30 minutes until golden brown on top and set within.
7. Take out the bread and allow cooling for a few minutes.
8. Slice and serve.

PER SERVING

Cal 227| Fat 15.3g| Carbs 15g| Protein 9g

Radish Hash Browns
Prep time: 10 minutes | Cook time: 10 minutes | Serves 8

- 2 pounds radishes, trimmed
- 4 tablespoons olive oil
- 1 large egg, whisked
- ⅛ teaspoon salt
- ⅛ teaspoon black pepper

1. Shred radishes using a food processor or hand grater and squeeze out extra moisture using cheesecloth or clean dish towel.
2. In a medium skillet over medium heat, heat oil. Add radishes and stir often. Sauté 20–30 minutes until golden. Remove from heat and place into a medium bowl.
3. Stir whisked egg into bowl with salt and pepper.
4. Form ten small pancakes. Add back to hot skillet. Heat 3-5 minutes on each side until solid and brown.
5. Serve warm.

PER SERVING

Calories: 63 | Fat: 6g | Protein: 1g | Sodium: 58mg| Fiber: 1g |Carbohydrates: 2g | Net Carbs: 1g | Sugar: 1g

Almond Butter Pancakes
Prep time: 5 minutes | Cook time:10 minutes |Serves 1

- Nonstick cooking spray
- 2 tablespoons almond butter
- ¼ cup unsweetened cashew milk
- 5 or 6 drops liquid stevia
- 1 tablespoon ground flaxseed
- 1 tablespoon coconut flour
- ½ teaspoon baking powder
- ½ teaspoon ground cinnamon
- 2 tablespoons grass-fed butter

1. Spray a skillet with nonstick cooking spray.
2. In a small bowl, combine the almond butter, cashew milk, and stevia.
3. In a separate small bowl, combine the flaxseed, coconut flour, baking powder, and cinnamon. Mix well.
4. Pour the almond-butter-and-milk mixture into the flour mixture and stir until well blended.
5. Allow the batter to sit for 3 to 4 minutes to thicken.
6. Heat the skillet over medium-high heat. When hot, pour the batter into 3- to 4-inch circles and cook for about 4 minutes.
7. Flip the pancakes and cook for an additional 2 minutes.
8. Top with the grass-fed butter and enjoy.

PER SERVING

Calories: 573 | Fat: 55g | Protein: 9g | Total Carbs: 11g | Net Carbs: 4g | Fiber: 7g | Sugar: 1g | Sodium: 288mg | Macros: Fat: 86% | Protein: 6% | Carbs: 8%

Zucchini Chocolate Muffins

Prep time: 5 minutes | Cook time:15 minutes | Serves 4

- 3 eggs, beaten
- 2 cups shredded zucchini
- ½ cup cacao powder
- ½ cup coconut oil, slightly melted
- 1 teaspoon vanilla extract
- ⅓ cup granulated erythritol
- 2 tablespoons low-carb dark chocolate chips

1. Preheat the oven to 250°F.
2. Grease the cups of a muffin tin (or use liners).
3. In a medium bowl, mix together the eggs, zucchini, cacao powder, coconut oil, vanilla, and erythritol.
4. Pour the batter evenly into the 12 muffin cups.
5. Sprinkle the chocolate chips on the tops of the muffins.
6. Bake for about 15 minutes, or until a knife inserted into the middle of a muffin comes out clean.
7. Transfer the muffins to a cooling rack.

PER SERVING

Calories: 379 | Fat: 35g | Protein: 7g | Total Carbs: 9g | Net Carbs: 5g | Fiber: 4g | Sugar: 1g | Sodium: 54mg; Erythritol carbs: 6g Macros: Fat: 83% | Protein: 7% | Carbs: 10%

Choco-Berry Smoothie

Prep time: 5 minutes | Cook time:5 minutes | Serves 3

- 1 tbsp poppy seeds
- 2 cups soy milk
- 2 cups blackberries
- 2 tbsp pure maple syrup
- 2 tbsp cocoa powder

1. Submerge poppy seeds in soy milk and let sit for 5 minutes.
2. Transfer to a food processor and add soy milk, blackberries, maple syrup, and cocoa powder.
3. Blitz until smooth.
4. Serve right away in glasses.
5. Enjoy!

PER SERVING

Cal 288 | Fat 8g | Carbs 47g | Protein 12g | Fiber: 4g

Green Monster Smoothie

Prep time: 3 minutes | Cook time: 5 minutes | Serves 1

- 1 cup ice
- 1 cup chopped fresh spinach
- ½ cup fresh raspberries
- 2 (1-gram) packets 0g net carb sweetener

1. 1 cup unsweetened almond milk (or dairy alternative milk of your choice)
2. Pulse all ingredients in a food processor or blender 30–60 seconds until ice is blended.

PER SERVING

Calories: 67 | Fat: 3g | Protein: 3g | Sodium: 203mg | Fiber: 6g | Carbohydrates: 10g | Net Carbs: 4g | Sugar: 3g

Orange-Carrot Muffins with Cherries

Prep time:10 minutes | Cook time:35 minutes | Serves 6

- 1 tsp avocado oil
- 2 tbsp almond butter
- ¼ cup non-dairy milk
- 1 orange, peeled
- 1 carrot, coarsely chopped
- 2 tbsp chopped dried cherries
- 3 tbsp molasses
- 2 tbsp ground flaxseed
- 1 tsp apple cider vinegar
- 1 tsp pure vanilla extract
- ½ tsp ground cinnamon
- ½ tsp ground ginger
- ¼ tsp ground nutmeg
- ¼ tsp allspice
- ¾ cup whole-wheat flour
- 1 tsp baking powder
- ½ tsp baking soda
- ½ cup rolled oats
- 2 tbsp raisins
- 2 tbsp sunflower seeds

1. Preheat your oven to 350°F.
2. Grease 6 muffin cups with avocado oil.
3. In a food processor, add the almond butter, milk, orange, carrot, cherries, molasses, flaxseed, vinegar, vanilla, cinnamon, ginger, nutmeg, and allspice and blend until smooth.
4. In a bowl, combine the flour, baking powder, and baking soda.
5. Fold in the wet mixture and gently stir to combine.
6. Mix in the oats, raisins, and sunflower seeds.
7. Divide the batter between muffin cups.
8. Put in a baking tray and bake for 30 minutes.

PER SERVING

Cal 210 | Fat 5g | Carbs 36.6g | Protein 5.3g

Berry Quinoa Bowl

Prep time: 5 minutes | Cook time:5 minutes | Serves 4

- 3 cups cooked quinoa
- 2 cups almond milk
- 2 bananas, sliced
- 2 cups berries
- ½ cup chopped hazelnuts
- ¼ cup maple syrup

1. In a large bowl, combine the quinoa, milk, banana, raspberries, blueberries, and hazelnuts.
2. Divide between serving bowls and top with maple syrup to serve.

PER SERVING

Cal 960| Fat 42g| Carbs 128g| Protein 23g

Broccoli Quiche

Prep time: 10 minutes | Cook time:30 minutes |Serves 2

- Nonstick cooking spray
- 1 egg, plus 5 egg whites
- ½ cup plain nonfat Greek yogurt
- 1 teaspoon salt
- ¼ teaspoon freshly ground black pepper
- 1 tablespoon minced garlic
- 1 cup broccoli florets
- 1 cup shredded cheddar cheese

1. Preheat the oven to 400°F. Spray a 9-inch pie dish with cooking spray.
2. In a medium bowl, mix together the egg, egg whites, Greek yogurt, salt, pepper, and garlic.
3. Fold in the broccoli and cheddar cheese.
4. Pour the mixture into the prepared pie dish and bake for 30 minutes, or until the eggs are set.
5. Remove the quiche from the oven and allow it to cool for a few minutes before serving.

PER SERVING

Calories: 352 | Fat: 21g | Protein: 33g | Total Carbs: 8g | Net Carbs: 7g | Fiber: 1g | Sugar: 3g | Sodium: 1663mg | Macros: Fat: 54% | Protein: 38% | Carbs: 8%

Matcha Smoothie with Berries

Prep time: 5 minutes | Cook time:5 minutes | Serves 2

- 2 cups almond milk
- 2 cups blueberries
- 1 banana, chopped
- ¼ tsp ground cinnamon
- 1 tbsp chia seeds
- 1 tbsp Matcha powder
- ¼ tsp ground ginger

1. Place the almond milk, blueberries, banana, cinnamon, chia seeds, matcha powder, and ginger in a blender and pulse until smooth.
2. Serve right away.
3. Enjoy!

PER SERVING

Cal 210| Fat 6g| Carbs 30g| Protein 9g

Counterfeit Bagels

Prep time: 15 minutes | Cook time: 17 minutes | Serves 10

- 1½ cups blanched almond flour
- 1 tablespoon baking powder
- 2½ cups shredded whole milk mozzarella cheese
- 2 ounces full-fat cream cheese, softened
- 2 large eggs, whisked
- 2 tablespoons Everything but the Bagel seasoning
- 1 tablespoon unsalted butter, melted

1. Preheat oven to 400°F. Line a baking sheet with parchment paper.
2. In a small bowl, mix almond flour and baking powder.
3. In a medium microwave-safe bowl, mix mozzarella cheese, cream cheese, and whisked eggs.
4. Microwave cheese mixture 1 minute. Stir and microwave again 30 seconds. Let mixture cool until okay to handle.
5. Combine dry ingredients into cheese mixture. Work quickly, stirring with a sturdy spatula or bamboo spoon to create dough. Shape dough into approximately ¾"-thick snakes, and then form into ten bagels.
6. Place bagels on prepared baking sheet and sprinkle tops with seasoning. Bake 15 minutes until browning on top.
7. Remove bagels from oven, brush with melted butter, and serve.

PER SERVING

Calories: 236 | Fat: 18g | Protein: 11g | Sodium: 548mg| Fiber: 2g |Carbohydrates: 5g | Net Carbs: 3g | Sugar: 1g

Starbucks Egg Bites

Prep time: 5 minutes | Cook time: 30 minutes | Serves 6

- 5 large eggs, whisked
- 1 cup shredded Swiss cheese
- 1 cup full-fat cottage cheese
- ⅛ teaspoon salt
- ⅛ teaspoon black pepper
- 2 strips no-sugar-added bacon, cooked and crumbled

1. Preheat oven to 350°F.
2. In a large bowl, whisk together eggs, Swiss cheese, cottage cheese, salt, and pepper.
3. Pour six equal amounts of mixture into well-greased muffin tins (or use cupcake liners).
4. Top with bacon bits.
5. Bake 30 minutes until eggs are completely cooked.
6. Remove Starbucks Egg Bites from oven and serve warm.

PER SERVING

Calories: 182 | Fat: 11g | Protein: 16g | Sodium: 321mg|
Fiber: 0g |Carbohydrates: 3g | Net Carbs: 3g | Sugar: 1g

Amazing Banana Oat Pancakes

Prep time: 5 minutes | Cook time:10 minutes | Serves 2

- 2 tsp ground cinnamon
- 2 eggs
- 1 egg white
- 1 banana
- 1 cup rolled oats
- 1 tbsp coconut oil
- 1 tsp vanilla extract
- ½ tsp sea salt

1. Place the oats in a food processor and pulse until it gets a coarse flour.
2. Add in cinnamon, eggs, egg white, banana, vanilla, and salt and blitz until smooth.
3. Brush a frying pan with some coconut oil.
4. Cook your pancakes for 4 minutes until the edges begin to brown.
5. Flip and cook your pancake on the other side for about 3 minutes more.
6. Serve warm with your favorite topping.
7. Enjoy!

PER SERVING

Cal 305| Fat 16g| Carbs 18g| Protein 16g

Maple Coconut Pancakes

Prep time: 5 minutes | Cook time:50 minutes | Serves 4

- ½ cup coconut flour
- 4 eggs
- 1 cup coconut milk
- 1 tbsp pure maple syrup
- 1 tsp vanilla extract
- 1 tbsp melted coconut oil
- 1 tsp baking soda
- ½ tsp sea salt

1. Beat the eggs, coconut milk, maple syrup, vanilla, and coconut oil in a large bowl.
2. Stir to combine.
3. Put the coconut flour, baking soda, and salt in a separate bowl| mix well.
4. Add the egg mixture and whisk the batter well until smooth and no lump.
5. Heat a greased nonstick skillet over medium heat and cook your pancakes until the edges begin to brown.
6. Flip halfway through the cooking time.
7. Serve immediately.

PER SERVING

Cal 190| Fat 10g| Carbs 15g| Protein 8g

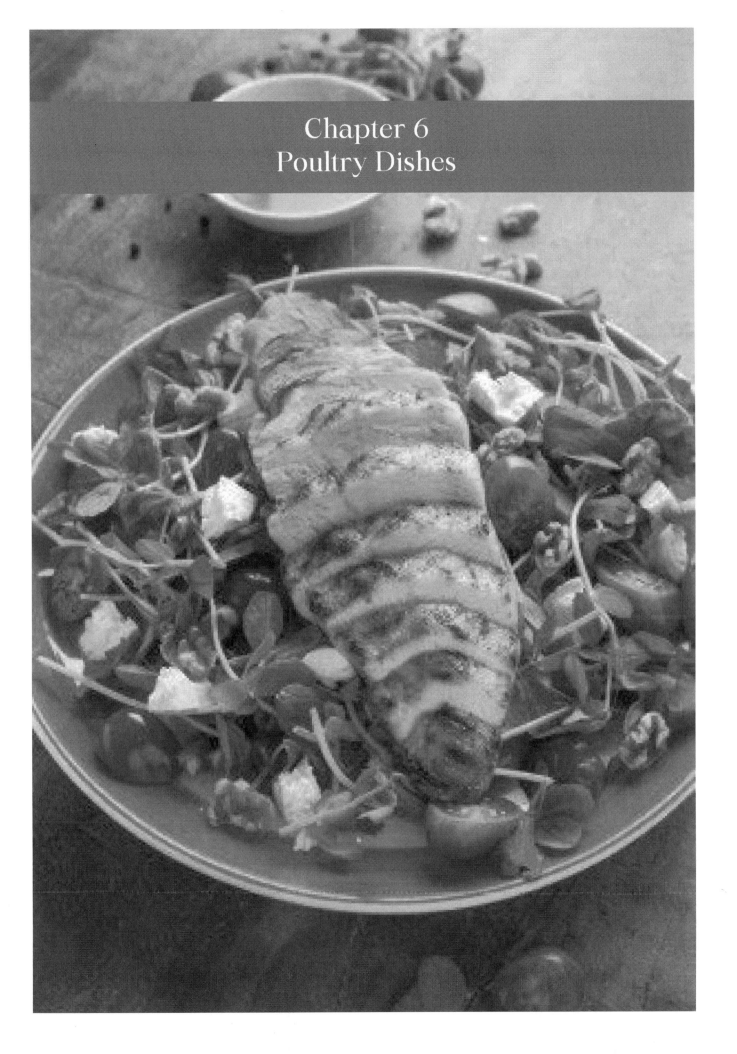

Chapter 6
Poultry Dishes

Italian-Style Chicken

Prep time: 5 minutes | Cook time:20 minutes | Serves 4

- 1 tbsp Italian seasoning
- 2 tbsp parsley, chopped
- 4 chicken breast halves
- 1 tsp garlic powder
- 2 tbsp olive oil
- 1 zucchini, chopped
- 2 cups cherry tomatoes
- ½ cup sliced green olives
- ¼ cup dry white wine

1. Pound the chicken breasts with a rolling pin to ½-inch thickness.
2. Sprinkle them with Italian seasoning and garlic powder.
3. Warm the olive oil in a skillet over medium heat and place in the breasts.
4. Sear for 14-20 minutes on all sides until slightly browned.
5. Set aside covered with foil.
6. Place the zucchini, tomatoes, and olives in the skillet and cook for 4 minutes until the zucchini is tender.
7. Pour in wine and scrape any brown bits from the bottom and simmer for 1 minute.
8. Add the chicken back to the pot and gently stir to coat in the sauce.
9. Garnish with parsley.

PER SERVING

Cal 170| Fat 12g| Carbs 9g| Protein 2g

Chicken-Basil Alfredo With Shirataki Noodles

Prep time: 10 minutes | Cook time: 15 minutes | Serves 2

FOR THE NOODLES

- 1 (7-ounce) package Miracle Noodle Fettuccini Shirataki Noodles
- For The Sauce
- 1 tablespoon olive oil
- 4 ounces cooked shredded chicken (I usually use a store-bought rotisserie chicken)
- Pink Himalayan salt
- Freshly ground black pepper
- 1 cup Alfredo Sauce, or any brand you like
- ¼ cup grated Parmesan cheese
- 2 tablespoons chopped fresh basil leaves

TO MAKE THE NOODLES

1. In a colander, rinse the noodles with cold water (shirataki noodles naturally have a smell, and rinsing with cold water will help remove this).
2. Fill a large saucepan with water and bring to a boil over high heat. Add the noodles and boil for 2 minutes. Drain.
3. Transfer the noodles to a large, dry skillet over medium-low heat to evaporate any moisture. Do not grease the skillet; it must be dry. Transfer the noodles to a plate and set aside.

TO MAKE THE SAUCE

1. In the saucepan over medium heat, heat the olive oil. Add the cooked chicken. Season with pink Himalayan salt and pepper.
2. Pour the Alfredo sauce over the chicken, and cook until warm. Season with more pink Himalayan salt and pepper.
3. Add the dried noodles to the sauce mixture, and toss until combined.
4. Divide the pasta between two plates, top each with the Parmesan cheese and chopped basil, and serve.

PER SERVING

Calories: 673 | Total Fat: 61g | Carbs: 4g | Net Carbs: 4g | Fiber: 0g | Protein: 29g

Braised Chicken Thighs With Kalamata Olives

Prep time: 10 minutes | Cook time: 40 minutes | Serves 2

- 4 chicken thighs, skin on
- Pink Himalayan salt
- Freshly ground black pepper
- 2 tablespoons ghee
- ½ cup chicken broth
- 1 lemon, ½ sliced and ½ juiced
- ½ cup pitted Kalamata olives
- 2 tablespoons butter

1. Preheat the oven to 375°F.
2. Pat the chicken thighs dry with paper towels, and season with pink Himalayan salt and pepper.
3. In a medium oven-safe skillet or high-sided baking dish over medium-high heat, melt the ghee. When the ghee has melted and is hot, add the chicken thighs, skin-side down, and leave them for about 8 minutes, or until the skin is brown and crispy.
4. Flip the chicken and cook for 2 minutes on the second side. Around the chicken thighs, pour in the chicken broth, and add the lemon slices, lemon juice, and olives.
5. Bake in the oven for about 30 minutes, until the chicken is cooked through.
6. Add the butter to the broth mixture.
7. Divide the chicken and olives between two plates and serve.

PER SERVING

Calories: 567 | Total Fat: 47g | Carbs: 4g | Net Carbs: 2g | Fiber: 2g | Protein: 33g

Buttery Garlic Chicken

Prep time: 5 minutes | Cook time: 40 minutes | Serves 2

- 2 tablespoons ghee, melted
- 2 boneless skinless chicken breasts
- Pink Himalayan salt
- Freshly ground black pepper
- 1 tablespoon dried Italian seasoning
- 4 tablespoons butter
- 2 garlic cloves, minced
- ¼ cup grated Parmesan cheese

1. Preheat the oven to 375°F. Choose a baking dish that is large enough to hold both chicken breasts and coat it with the ghee.
2. Pat dry the chicken breasts and season with pink Himalayan salt, pepper, and Italian seasoning. Place the chicken in the baking dish.
3. In a medium skillet over medium heat, melt the butter. Add the minced garlic, and cook for about 5 minutes. You want the garlic very lightly browned but not burned.
4. Remove the butter-garlic mixture from the heat, and pour it over the chicken breasts.

5. Roast the chicken in the oven for 30 to 35 minutes, until cooked through. Sprinkle some of the Parmesan cheese on top of each chicken breast. Let the chicken rest in the baking dish for 5 minutes.
6. Divide the chicken between two plates, spoon the butter sauce over the chicken, and serve.

PER SERVING

Calories: 642 | Total Fat: 45g | Carbs: 2g | Net Carbs: 2g | Fiber: 0g | Protein: 57g

Italian Turkey Meatballs

Prep time: 5 minutes | Cook time:7 hours 10 minutes | Serves 4

- 1 spaghetti squash, halved lengthwise, scoop out seeds
- 1 (14-oz) can diced tomatoes
- ½ tsp garlic powder
- ½ tsp dried oregano
- ½ tsp sea salt
- 1 large egg, whisked
- ½ white onion, minced
- 1 lb ground turkey
- Sea salt and pepper to taste
- ½ tsp dried basil
- 1 cup arugula

1. Pour the diced tomatoes into your slow cooker.
2. Sprinkle with garlic powder, oregano, and salt.
3. Put in the squash halves, cut-side down.
4. In a medium bowl, mix together the turkey, egg, onion, salt, pepper, and basil.
5. Shape the turkey mixture into balls and place them in the slow cooker around the spaghetti squash.
6. Cover the cooker and set to "Low".
7. Cook for 7 hours.
8. Transfer the squash to a work surface and use a fork to shred it into spaghetti-like strands.
9. Combine the strands with the tomato sauce, top with the meatballs and arugula, and serve.

PER SERVING

Cal 250| Fat 8g| Carbs 21g| Protein 23g

Cheesy Bacon And Broccoli Chicken

Prep time: 10 minutes | Cook time: 1 hour | Serves 2

- 2 tablespoons ghee
- 2 boneless skinless chicken breasts
- Pink Himalayan salt
- Freshly ground black pepper
- 4 bacon slices
- 6 ounces cream cheese, at room temperature
- 2 cups frozen broccoli florets, thawed
- ½ cup shredded Cheddar cheese

1. Preheat the oven to 375°F.
2. Choose a baking dish that is large enough to hold both chicken breasts and coat it with the ghee.
3. Pat dry the chicken breasts with a paper towel, and season with pink Himalayan salt and pepper.
4. Place the chicken breasts and the bacon slices in the baking dish, and bake for 25 minutes.
5. Transfer the chicken to a cutting board and use two forks to shred it. Season it again with pink Himalayan salt and pepper.
6. Place the bacon on a paper towel–lined plate to crisp up, and then crumble it.
7. In a medium bowl, mix to combine the cream cheese, shredded chicken, broccoli, and half of the bacon crumbles. Transfer the chicken mixture to the baking dish, and top with the Cheddar and the remaining half of the bacon crumbles.
8. Bake until the cheese is bubbling and browned, about 35 minutes, and serve.

PER SERVING

Calories: 935 | Total Fat: 66g | Carbs: 10g | Net Carbs: 8g | Fiber: 3g | Protein: 75g

Classic Chicken Cacciatore

Prep time: 5 minutes | Cook time:25 minutes | Serves 4

- 2 tbsp red wine
- 2 rosemary sprigs, chopped
- 2 tbsp olive oil
- 4 chicken breasts, cubed
- 2 (28-oz) cans diced tomatoes
- ½ cup black olives, chopped
- 2 garlic cloves, minced
- 1 shallot, chopped
- Sea salt and pepper to taste

1. Warm the olive oil in a skillet over medium heat.
2. Add in the chicken and cook for 6-8 minutes, stirring periodically to promote even cooking.
3. Stir in shallot and garlic and sauté for further 3 minutes.
4. Pour in the red wine, tomatoes, olives, salt, and pepper and simmer for 8-10 minutes.
5. Scatter with chopped rosemary and serve.

PER SERVING

Cal 310| Fat 12g| Carbs 35g| Protein 14g

Parmesan Baked Chicken

Prep time: 5 minutes | Cook time: 20 minutes | Serves 2

- 2 tablespoons ghee
- 2 boneless skinless chicken breasts
- Pink Himalayan salt
- Freshly ground black pepper
- ½ cup mayonnaise
- ¼ cup grated Parmesan cheese
- 1 tablespoon dried Italian seasoning
- ¼ cup crushed pork rinds

1. Preheat the oven to 425°F. Choose a baking dish that is large enough to hold both chicken breasts and coat it with the ghee.
2. Pat dry the chicken breasts with a paper towel, season with pink Himalayan salt and pepper, and place in the prepared baking dish.
3. In a small bowl, mix to combine the mayonnaise, Parmesan cheese, and Italian seasoning.
4. Slather the mayonnaise mixture evenly over the chicken breasts, and sprinkle the crushed pork rinds on top of the mayonnaise mixture.
5. Bake until the topping is browned, about 20 minutes, and serve.

PER SERVING

Calories: 850 | Total Fat: 67g | Carbs: 2g | Net Carbs: 2g | Fiber: 0g | Protein: 60g

Sicilian Chicken Bake

Prep time: 5 minutes | Cook time:25 minutes | Serves 4

- 1 cup sliced cremini mushrooms
- 4 garlic cloves, minced
- 4 chicken breasts
- 2 tbsp avocado oil
- 1 cup chopped spinach
- 1 fennel bulb, sliced
- 20 cherry tomatoes, halved
- ½ cup chopped fresh basil
- ½ red onion, thinly sliced
- 2 tsp balsamic vinegar

1. Preheat your oven to 400°F.
2. Arrange the chicken breasts on a baking dish and brush them generously with avocado oil.
3. Mix together the mushrooms, spinach, fennel, tomatoes, basil, red onion, garlic, and balsamic vinegar in a medium bowl and toss to combine.
4. Top the breasts with the vegetable mixture.
5. Bake in the oven for about 20 minutes, or until the juices run clear when pierced with a fork.
6. Allow the chicken to rest for 5-10 minutes before slicing.
7. Serve and enjoy!

PER SERVING

Cal 225| Fat 8g| Carbs 7g| Protein 27g

Aromatic Turkey with Mushrooms

Prep time: 5 minutes | Cook time: 4 hours 10 minutes | Serves 4

- 2 cups button mushrooms, sliced
- 2 turkey thighs
- 1 red bell pepper, sliced
- 1 large onion, sliced
- 1 garlic clove, sliced
- 1 tbsp extra-virgin olive oil
- 1 rosemary sprig
- Sea salt and pepper to taste
- 2 cups chicken broth
- ½ cup dry red wine

1. Grease your slow cooker with olive oil.
2. Add the turkey thighs, bell pepper, mushrooms, onion, garlic, rosemary sprig, salt, and pepper.
3. Pour in the chicken broth and wine.
4. Cover and cook on "High" for 4 hours.
5. Remove and discard the rosemary sprig.
6. Use a slotted spoon to transfer the thighs to a plate and allow them to cool for several minutes for easier handling.
7. Cut the meat from the bones, stir the meat into the mushrooms, and serve.

PER SERVING

Cal 275| Fat 9g| Carbs 3g| Protein 42g

Chicken a la Tuscana

Prep time: 5 minutes | Cook time: 20 minutes | Serves 4

- 2 cups cherry tomatoes
- 4 chicken breast halves
- 1 tsp garlic powder
- Sea salt and pepper to taste
- 2 tbsp extra-virgin olive oil
- ½ cup sliced green olives
- 1 eggplant, chopped
- ¼ cup dry white wine

1. Pound the chicken breasts with a meat tenderizer until half an inch thick.
2. Rub them with garlic powder, salt, and ground black pepper.
3. Warm the olive oil in a skillet over medium heat.
4. Add the chicken and cook for 14-16 minutes, flipping halfway through the cooking time.
5. Transfer to a plate and cover with aluminum foil.
6. Add the tomatoes, olives, and eggplant to the skillet and sauté for 4 minutes or until the vegetables are soft.
7. Add the white wine to the skillet and simmer for 1 minute.
8. Remove the aluminum foil and top the chicken with the vegetables and their juices, then serve warm.

PER SERVING

Cal 170| Fat 10g| Carbs 8g| Protein 7g

Chicken Skewers With Peanut Sauce

Prep time: 10 minutes | Cook time: 15 minutes | Serves 2

- 1 pound boneless skinless chicken breast, cut into chunks
- 3 tablespoons soy sauce (or coconut aminos), divided
- ½ teaspoon Sriracha sauce, plus ¼ teaspoon
- 3 teaspoons toasted sesame oil, divided
- Ghee, for oiling
- 2 tablespoons peanut butter
- Pink Himalayan salt
- Freshly ground black pepper

1. In a large zip-top bag, combine the chicken chunks with 2 tablespoons of soy sauce, ½ teaspoon of Sriracha sauce, and 2 teaspoons of sesame oil. Seal the bag, and let the chicken marinate for an hour or so in the refrigerator or up to overnight.
2. If you are using wood 8-inch skewers, soak them in water for 30 minutes before using.
3. I like to use my grill pan for the skewers, because I don't have an outdoor grill. If you don't have a grill pan, you can use a large skillet. Preheat your grill pan or grill to low. Oil the grill pan with ghee.
4. Thread the chicken chunks onto the skewers.
5. Cook the skewers over low heat for 10 to 15 minutes, flipping halfway through.
6. Meanwhile, mix the peanut dipping sauce. Stir together the remaining 1 tablespoon of soy sauce, ¼ teaspoon of Sriracha sauce, 1 teaspoon of sesame oil, and the peanut butter. Season with pink Himalayan salt and pepper.
7. Serve the chicken skewers with a small dish of the peanut sauce.

PER SERVING

Calories: 586 | Total Fat: 29g | Carbs: 6g | Net Carbs: 5g | Fiber: 1g | Protein: 75g

Cheesy Broccoli-Stuffed Chicken

Prep time: 15 minutes | Cook time: 25 minutes | Serves 4

FOR THE FILLING:

- 2 cups chopped cooked broccoli
- ½ cup mascarpone cheese (4 ounces)
- 3 tablespoons grated Parmesan cheese
- ½ teaspoon kosher salt
- ¼ teaspoon ground black pepper
- ⅛ teaspoon garlic powder
- ⅛ teaspoon ground nutmeg
- 4 (6-ounce) chicken cutlets, pounded to ½-inch thickness
- ½ cup Keto Breadcrumbs
- 2 tablespoons grated Parmesan cheese
- 1 teaspoon dried parsley leaves
- ½ teaspoon kosher salt
- ¼ teaspoon ground black pepper
- ⅛ teaspoon garlic powder
- 1 large egg, beaten

1. Preheat the oven to 375°F. Line a 15 by 10-inch sheet pan with parchment paper.
2. Make the filling: Put the cooked broccoli, mascarpone, Parmesan cheese, salt, pepper, garlic powder, and nutmeg in a medium-sized bowl and mix well.
3. Lay the chicken cutlets on a cutting board and spoon about ½ cup of the filling onto the center of each cutlet. Roll the chicken up around the filling and secure each cutlet with a toothpick.
4. Place the breadcrumbs, Parmesan cheese, parsley, salt, pepper, and garlic powder in a small bowl and mix well. Dip the stuffed cutlets into the beaten egg, then into the seasoned breadcrumbs. Place the breaded cutlets on the lined sheet pan and sprinkle any remaining breadcrumbs over the top of the chicken.
5. Bake for 25 minutes, or until the center of the cutlets reads 165°F on a meat thermometer. Serve immediately.

PER SERVING

Calories: 488 | Fat: 25g | Protein: 50g | Carbs: 4g | Fiber: 2g | Net Carbs: 2g

Chicken Larb

Prep time: 10 minutes | Cook time: 8 minutes | Serves 4

- 1 tablespoon coconut oil
- 1 pound ground chicken
- ½ cup thinly sliced red onions, plus more for garnish if desired
- 1 tablespoon peeled and minced fresh ginger
- 1 teaspoon minced garlic
- ½ teaspoon red pepper flakes
- 1 tablespoon fish sauce (no sugar added)
- 1 tablespoon wheat-free soy sauce
- 1 teaspoon Sriracha sauce, plus more for serving if desired
- 1 tablespoon lime juice
- For Serving/Garnish:
- Leaves from 1 large head or 2 small heads butter and/or leaf lettuce
- 2 cups Basic Cauliflower Rice, hot
- 2 tablespoons chopped fresh basil
- 2 tablespoons chopped fresh cilantro
- 2 tablespoons chopped fresh mint
- Lime wedges, for serving (optional)

1. Heat the coconut oil in a large sauté pan. Add the chicken, onions, ginger, garlic, and red pepper flakes and cook, stirring occasionally, for 5 minutes, or until fragrant.
2. Add the fish sauce, soy sauce, and Sriracha and cook for 3 more minutes, or until most of the liquid has been absorbed.
3. Remove from the heat and stir in the lime juice. Serve the chicken mixture over the lettuce leaves and cauliflower rice and garnish with the fresh herbs. If desired, top with a few extra slices of onion and serve with lime wedges and Sriracha on the side.

PER SERVING

Calories: 200 | Fat: 8g | Protein: 26g | Carbs: 6g | Fiber: 1g | Net Carbs: 5g

Tandoori Chicken Meatballs

Prep time: 10 minutes, plus 1 hour to chill | Cook time: 10 minutes | Makes 12 meatballs

- 1 pound ground chicken
- 2 tablespoons full-fat Greek yogurt
- 2 tablespoons minced red onions
- 2 teaspoons lemon juice
- 1 teaspoon kosher salt
- 1 teaspoon peeled and minced fresh ginger
- 1 teaspoon minced garlic
- 1 teaspoon paprika
- ½ teaspoon cayenne pepper
- ½ teaspoon garam masala
- ½ teaspoon ground cumin
- ½ teaspoon turmeric powder
- 1 large egg, beaten
- ½ cup superfine blanched almond flour
- 2 tablespoons avocado oil or other light-tasting oil, for the pan

1. Place all of the ingredients, except for the oil, in a medium-sized bowl and mix well. Chill for at least 1 hour or up to 24 hours to allow the flavors to come together.
2. Use your hands to form the chicken mixture into 12 meatballs, each about 2 inches in diameter.
3. Heat the oil in a large sauté pan over medium heat. Place the meatballs in the pan and cook for about 4 minutes per side, until golden brown and cooked through.
4. Meanwhile, turn on the oven to broil-high.
5. Transfer the meatballs to a sheet pan and broil in the oven for 2 to 3 minutes, until slightly charred on the outside.

PER SERVING

Calories: 355 | Fat: 27g | Protein: 24g | Carbs: 5g | Fiber: 2g | Net Carbs: 3g

Jerk Chicken

Prep time: 2 minutes | Cook time: 30 minutes | Serves 6

- 6 whole chicken legs (drumsticks and thighs)
- 2 tablespoons Jerk Seasoning
- 1½ teaspoons kosher salt
- ½ cup Easy Keto BBQ Sauce

1. Preheat a grill to medium heat.
2. Coat the chicken legs liberally with the jerk seasoning and salt. Grill the chicken for 20 minutes, turning occasionally.
3. Brush the BBQ sauce on the chicken and grill for 5 more minutes per side, or until a meat thermometer inserted in the thickest part of a thigh reads 165°F.

PER SERVING

Calories: 350 | Fat: 20g | Protein: 38g | Carbs: 3g | Fiber: 0.5g | Net Carbs: 2.5g

Chicken Cacciatore

Prep time: 10 minutes | Cook time: 45 minutes | Serves 8

- 8 bone-in, skin-on chicken thighs
- 1 teaspoon kosher salt
- ½ teaspoon ground black pepper
- 2 tablespoons extra-virgin olive oil
- 1 cup sliced red bell peppers
- 1 cup sliced yellow bell peppers
- ½ cup sliced yellow onions
- 1 tablespoon minced garlic
- ½ cup dry white wine
- 1 (28-ounce) can diced tomatoes
- ¾ cup chicken broth, store-bought or homemade
- 1 tablespoon capers, drained
- 1 teaspoon dried oregano leaves
- 2 tablespoons chopped fresh basil, for garnish
- 2 tablespoons chopped fresh parsley, for garnish

1. Season the chicken with the salt and pepper. Heat the olive oil in a large sauté pan over medium heat for 2 minutes. Brown the chicken on all sides, about 3 minutes per side. Remove the chicken from the pan and set aside.
2. Place the bell peppers, onions, and garlic in the same pan and cook until the peppers and onions begin to soften, about 5 minutes.
3. Add the wine and cook until reduced by half, about 2 minutes. Add the tomatoes, broth, capers, oregano, and chicken thighs to the pan. Simmer, uncovered, until the chicken is cooked through, about 30 minutes.
4. Remove the chicken to a platter. Increase the heat to high and cook the sauce for about 3 minutes, stirring constantly, until it has reduced and thickened slightly. Taste and season with more salt and pepper, if desired.
5. Pour the sauce over the chicken and garnish with the basil and parsley. Serve immediately.

PER SERVING

Calories: 430 | Fat: 26g | Protein: 37g | Carbs: 5.5g | Fiber: 1.5g | Net Carbs: 4g

Chicken Quesadilla

Prep time: 5 minutes | Cook time: 5 minutes | Serves 2

- 1 tablespoon olive oil
- 2 low-carbohydrate tortillas
- ½ cup shredded Mexican blend cheese
- 2 ounces shredded chicken (I usually use a store-bought rotisserie chicken)
- 1 teaspoon Tajín seasoning salt
- 2 tablespoons sour cream

1. In a large skillet over medium-high heat, heat the olive oil. Add a tortilla, then layer on top ¼ cup of cheese, the chicken, the Tajín seasoning, and the remaining ¼ cup of cheese. Top with the second tortilla.
2. Peek under the edge of the bottom tortilla to monitor how it is browning. Once the bottom tortilla gets golden and the cheese begins to melt, after about 2 minutes, flip the quesadilla over. The second side will cook faster, about 1 minute.
3. Once the second tortilla is crispy and golden, transfer the quesadilla to a cutting board and let sit for 2 minutes. Cut the quesadilla into 4 wedges using a pizza cutter or chef's knife.
4. Transfer half the quesadilla to each of two plates. Add 1 tablespoon of sour cream to each plate, and serve hot.

PER SERVING

Calories: 414 | Total Fat: 28g | Carbs: 24g | Net Carbs: 7g | Fiber: 17g | Protein: 26g

Cherry-Balsamic Chicken Breasts

Prep time: 5 minutes | Cook time:35 minutes | Serves 4

- 2 tbsp parsley, chopped
- 4 chicken breasts
- 2 scallions, sliced
- 2 tbsp coconut oil
- ¾ cup chicken broth
- 1 tbsp balsamic vinegar
- ½ cup dried cherries
- Sea salt and pepper to taste

1. Preheat your oven to 375°F.
2. Melt the coconut oil in a large skillet over medium heat.
3. Season the chicken with salt and pepper.
4. Place the chicken in the pan and brown it on both sides, 3 minutes per side.
5. Add the scallions, chicken broth, balsamic vinegar, and dried cherries.
6. Cover with an oven-proof lid or aluminum foil and place the pan in the preheated oven.
7. Bake for 20 minutes, or until the chicken is cooked through.
8. Top with parsley.

PER SERVING

Cal 380| Fat 15g| Carbs 17g| Protein 42g

Garlic-Parmesan Chicken Wings

Prep time: 10 minutes | Cook time: 3 hours | Serves 2

- 8 tablespoons (1 stick) butter
- 2 garlic cloves, minced
- 1 tablespoon dried Italian seasoning
- ¼ cup grated Parmesan cheese, plus ½ cup
- Pink Himalayan salt
- Freshly ground black pepper
- 1 pound chicken wings

1. With the crock insert in place, preheat the slow cooker to high. Line a baking sheet with aluminum foil or a silicone baking mat.
2. Put the butter, garlic, Italian seasoning, and ¼ cup of Parmesan cheese in the slow cooker, and season with pink Himalayan salt and pepper. Allow the butter to melt, and stir the ingredients until well mixed.
3. Add the chicken wings and stir until coated with the butter mixture.
4. Cover the slow cooker and cook for 2 hours and 45 minutes.
5. Preheat the broiler.
6. Transfer the wings to the prepared baking sheet, sprinkle the remaining ½ cup of Parmesan cheese over the wings, and cook under the broiler until crispy, about 5 minutes.
7. Serve hot.

PER SERVING

Calories: 738 | Total Fat: 66g | Carbs: 4g | Net Carbs: 4g | Fiber: 0g | Protein: 39g

Sumac Chicken Thighs

Prep time: 5 minutes | Cook time:50 minutes | Serves 4

- 6 bone-in chicken thighs
- 2 sweet potatoes, cubed
- 2 tbsp extra-virgin olive oil
- 2 shallots, sliced thin
- Sea salt and pepper to taste
- 1 tsp sumac
- ½ tsp ground cinnamon
- 1 cup chicken broth

1. Preheat your oven to 425°F.
2. In a large baking dish, stir together the oil, shallots, salt, cumin, cinnamon, pepper, and chicken broth.
3. Add the chicken and sweet potatoes.
4. Stir to coat with the spices.
5. Place the dish in the preheated oven and bake for 35-45 minutes, or until the chicken is cooked through and the sweet potatoes are tender.
6. Serve.

PER SERVING

Cal 520| Fat 32g| Carbs 22g| Protein 32g

Broccoli & Chicken Stir-Fry
Prep time: 5 minutes | Cook time:15 minutes | Serves 4

- 2 cups broccoli florets
- 1 ½ lb chicken breasts, cubed
- ½ onion, chopped
- Sea salt and pepper to taste
- 3 tbsp extra-virgin olive oil
- 3 garlic cloves, minced

1. Warm the olive oil in a skillet over medium heat.
2. Add the broccoli, chicken, garlic, and onion and stir-fry for about 8 minutes, or until the chicken is golden browned and cooked through.
3. Season with salt and pepper.
4. Serve.

PER SERVING

Cal 345| Fat 13g| Carbs 4g| Protein 13g

Baked Basil Chicken
Prep time: 5 minutes | Cook time:40 minutes | Serves 4

- 2 garlic cloves, sliced
- 1 white onion, chopped
- 14 oz tomatoes, chopped
- 2 tbsp chopped rosemary
- Sea salt and pepper to taste
- 4 skinless chicken thighs
- 1 lb peeled pumpkin, cubed
- 1 tbsp extra virgin olive oil
- 2 tbsp basil leaves
- Preheat your oven to 375°F.

1. Warm the olive oil in a skillet over medium heat.
2. Add the garlic and onion and sauté for 5 minutes or until fragrant.
3. Add the tomatoes, rosemary, salt, and pepper and cook for 15 minutes or until slightly thickened.
4. Arrange the chicken thighs and pumpkin cubes on a baking sheet, then pour the mixture in the skillet over the chicken and sweet potatoes.
5. Stir to coat well.
6. Pour in enough water to cover the chicken and sweet potatoes.
7. Bake in for 20 minutes.
8. Top with basil.

PER SERVING

Cal 295| Fat 9g| Carbs 32g| Protein 21g

Rosemary Turkey with Mushrooms
Prep time: 5 minutes | Cook time:15 minutes | Serves 4

- 1 ½ lb boneless, skinless turkey breasts, cubed
- 3 tbsp olive oil
- 1 cup mushrooms, sliced
- 1 onion, chopped
- 2 tbsp chopped rosemary
- Sea salt and pepper to taste
- 3 garlic cloves, minced

1. Warm the olive oil in a skillet over medium heat.
2. Add the mushrooms, garlic, onion, turkey, salt, and pepper and stir-fry for 7-10 minutes until the meat is cooked through and the veggies are tender.
3. Garnish with rosemary.
4. Serve.

PER SERVING

Cal 310| Fat 15g| Carbs 16g| Protein 3g

Holiday Turkey
Prep time: 5 minutes | Cook time: 6 hours 10 minutes| Serves 4

- 1 lb turkey breast strips
- 1 celery stalk, minced
- 1 carrot, minced
- 1 shallot, diced
- ½ red bell pepper, chopped
- 1 tbsp extra-virgin olive oil
- 6 tbsp tomato paste
- 2 tbsp apple cider vinegar
- 1 tbsp pure maple syrup
- 1 tsp Dijon mustard
- 1 tsp chili powder
- ½ tsp garlic powder
- ½ tsp sea salt
- ½ tsp dried oregano

1. Blend the olive oil, turkey, celery, carrot, shallot, red bell pepper, tomato paste, vinegar, maple syrup, mustard, chili powder, garlic powder, salt, and oregano in your slow cooker.
2. Using a large spoon, break up the turkey into smaller chunks as it combines with the other ingredients.
3. Cover the cooker and set to "Low".
4. Cook for 6 hours.

PER SERVING

Cal 250| Fat 12g| Carbs 13g| Protein 23g

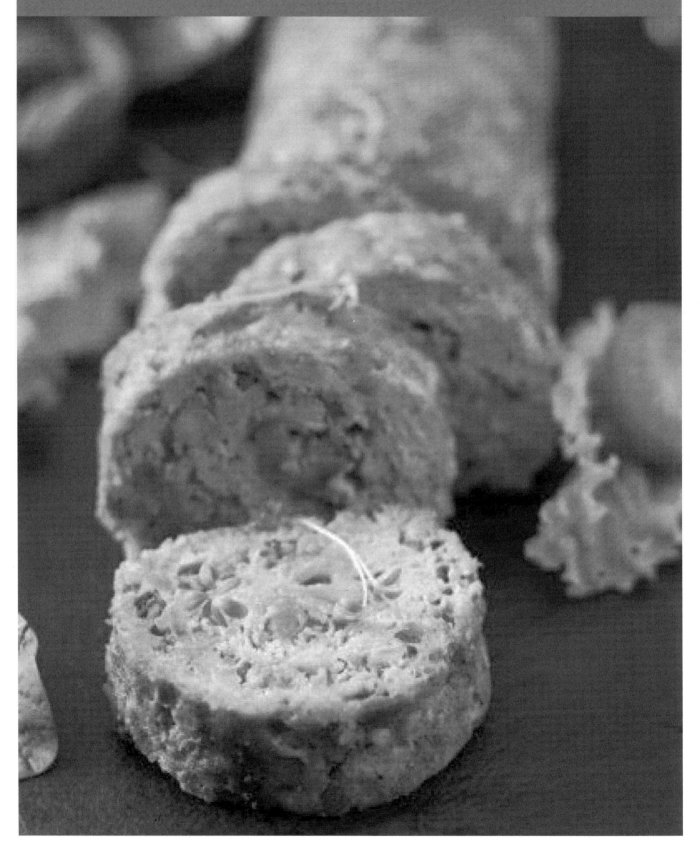

Chapter 7
Meat Dishes

Creamy Beef Tenderloin Marsala

Prep time: 5 minutes | Cook time:20 minutes | Serves 4

- 4 beef tenderloin fillets
- Sea salt and pepper to taste
- 2 tbsp olive oil
- 1 shallot, finely minced
- ½ cup Marsala wine
- 2 cups fresh blueberries
- 3 tbsp cold butter, cubed
- Pound the beef with a rolling pin to ¾-inch thickness.
- Sprinkle with salt and pepper.

1. Warm the olive oil in a skillet over medium heat.
2. Add the beef and brown for 10 minutes on both sides.
3. Set aside covered with foil.
4. Place the shallot, Marsala wine, blueberries, salt, and pepper in the skillet, and using a wide spatula, scrape any brown bits from the bottom.
5. Bring to a simmer, then low the heat, and simmer for 4 minutes, until blueberries break down and the liquid has reduced by half.
6. Add in butter cubed, one piece at time, and put the beef back to the skillet| toss to coat.
7. Serve and enjoy!

PER SERVING

Cal 550| Fat 33g| Carbs 15g| Protein 2g

Tangy Beef Carnitas

Prep time: 5 minutes | Cook time:25 minutes | Serves 4

- 1 tsp cayenne pepper
- 1 tsp paprika
- ¼ cup fresh cilantro leaves
- 6 tbsp olive oil
- 4 garlic cloves, minced
- 1 jalapeño pepper, chopped
- 1½ lb beef flank steak
- Sea salt and pepper to taste
- 1 cup guacamole

1. Place cilantro, 4 tbsp of olive oil, garlic, cayenne pepper, paprika, and jalapeño in your food processor and pulse until it reaches a paste consistency.
2. Reserve 1 tbsp of the paste.
3. Rub the flank steak with the remaining paste.
4. Warm the remaining olive oil in a skillet over medium heat.
5. Sear the steak for 15 minutes on all sides until browned.
6. Remove the meat to a cutting board and let it cool for 5 minutes.
7. Cut it against the grain into ½-inch-thick slices.
8. Put the beef in a bowl and add the reserved garlic paste| toss to combine.
9. Serve with guacamole.

PER SERVING

Cal 720| Fat 53g| Carbs 13g| Protein 2g

Hot & Spicy Beef Chili

Prep time: 5 minutes | Cook time:20 minutes | Serves 4

- 2 tbsp olive oil
- 1 tsp dried Mexican oregano
- 1 lb ground beef
- 1 onion, chopped
- 2 (28-oz) cans diced tomatoes
- 2 (14-oz) cans kidney beans,
- 1 tbsp red chili powder
- 1 tsp garlic powder
- ½ tsp sea salt

1. Warm the olive oil in a heavy-bottomed pot over medium heat.
2. Then, brown the ground beef for 5 minutes, crumbling with a wide spatula.
3. Mix in tomatoes, Mexican oregano, kidney beans, red chili powder, garlic powder, and salt and bring to a simmer.
4. Let it cook, partially covered, for 10 minutes longer.
5. Serve warm.

PER SERVING

Cal 900| Fat 21g| Carbs 64g| Protein 18g

Bistecca Alla Fiorentina

Prep time: 10 minutes | Cook time:35 minutes | Serves 4

- 2 (1-inch-thick) bone-in porterhouse steaks, about 2 pounds
- 6 tablespoons good-quality olive oil, divided
- Sea salt, for seasoning
- Freshly ground black pepper, for seasoning
- ½ cup white wine
- 2 rosemary sprigs
- Lemon wedges, for serving

1. 1.Preheat the grill. Preheat the grill to high heat.
2. Prepare the steaks. Rub the steaks with 2 tablespoons of the olive oil and season them generously with salt and pepper.
3. Prepare the basting liquid. In a small bowl, stir together the white wine and the remaining 4 tablespoons of olive oil.
4. Grill the steaks. Using the rosemary sprigs as basters, baste the steaks on both sides with the wine mixture. Grill the steaks, flipping them once, until they're seared on both sides, 6 to 8 minutes in total (125°F internal temperature) for medium rare.
5. Serve. Let the steaks rest for 10 minutes, then divide them between four plates, and serve them with lemon wedges.

PER SERVING

Calories: 569 | Total Fat: 45g | Total Carbs: 0g | Fiber: 0g | Net Carbs: 0g | Sodium: 238mg | Protein: 35g

Spicy Fried Beef With Chiles

Prep time: 10 minutes | Cook time: 1 hour 45 minutes | Serves 4

- 1½ tablespoons minced garlic
- 1 tablespoon grated fresh ginger
- 1 shallot, finely chopped
- 1 teaspoon chili powder
- 1 teaspoon ground cinnamon
- 1 teaspoon ground cumin
- ½ teaspoon ground coriander
- Pinch cayenne pepper
- 1½ pounds beef chuck, cut into 1-inch chunks
- ¼ cup good-quality olive oil
- 1 onion, peeled and thinly sliced
- 1 red bell pepper, thinly sliced
- 1 habanero pepper, minced
- 1 cup Beef Bone Broth
- 1 cup shredded unsweetened coconut
- ½ cup sour cream

1. Marinate the beef. In a medium bowl, stir together the garlic, ginger, shallot, chili powder, cinnamon, cumin, coriander, and cayenne to form a paste. Add the beef to the bowl and massage the paste into the pieces of beef. Cover the bowl and marinate the beef in the refrigerator for at least 4 hours.
2. Brown the beef. In a large saucepan over medium-high heat, warm the olive oil. Add the beef to the pan and sauté it until it has browned, about 10 minutes in total.
3. Sauté the vegetables. Add the onion, red bell pepper, and habanero pepper to the pan and sauté until they're tender, about 4 minutes.
4. Braise the beef. Add the beef broth and bring the liquid to a boil, then reduce the heat to low and simmer until the beef is very tender and the liquid reduces, about 1½ hours. Add more broth if the beef is not tender enough.
5. Finish and serve. Stir in the coconut and serve the beef topped with the sour cream.

PER SERVING

Calories: 528 | Total Fat: 37g | Total Carbs: 8g | Fiber: 4g | Net Carbs: 4g | Sodium: 275mg | Protein: 41g

Grilled Skirt Steak With Jalapeño Compound Butter

Prep time: 10 minutes | Cook time: 10 minutes | Serves 4

- ¼ cup unsalted grass-fed butter, at room temperature
- ½ jalapeño pepper, seeded and minced very finely
- Zest and juice of ½ lime
- ½ teaspoon sea salt
- 4 (4-ounce) skirt steaks
- 1 tablespoon olive oil
- Sea salt, for seasoning
- Freshly ground black pepper, for seasoning

1. Make the compound butter. In a medium bowl, stir together the butter, jalapeño pepper, lime zest, lime juice, and salt until everything is well combined. Lay a piece of plastic wrap on a clean work surface and spoon the butter mixture into the middle. Form the butter into a log about 1 inch thick by folding the plastic wrap over the butter and twisting the two ends in opposite directions. Roll the butter log on the counter to smooth the edges and put it in the freezer until it's very firm, about 4 hours.
2. Grill the steak. Preheat the grill to high heat. Lightly oil the steaks with the olive oil and season them lightly with salt and pepper. Grill the steaks for about 5 minutes per side for medium (140°F internal temperature) or until they're done the way you like them.
3. Rest and serve. Let the steaks rest for 10 minutes and serve them sliced across the grain, topped with a thick slice of the compound butter.

PER SERVING

Calories: 404 Total Fat: 32g | Total Carbs: 0g | Fiber: 0g | Net Carbs: 0g | Sodium: 292mg | Protein: 29g

Chili Pork Ragout

Prep time: 5 minutes | Cook time: 8 hours 10 minutes | Serves 4

- 1 cup spinach, minced
- 1 lb pork tenderloin
- 1 yellow onion, diced
- 1 red bell pepper, diced
- 1 can diced tomatoes
- 2 tsp chili powder
- 1 tsp garlic powder
- ½ tsp ground cumin
- 1 tsp fennel seeds
- ¼ tsp red pepper flakes

1. Add the pork, onion, bell pepper, tomatoes, chili powder, garlic powder, cumin, fennel seeds, red pepper flakes, and spinach in your slow cooker.
2. Cover the cooker and set to "Low".
3. Cook for 7-8 hours.
4. Transfer the pork loin to a cutting board and shred with a fork.
5. Return it to the slow cooker, stir it into the sauce, and serve.

PER SERVING

Cal 290| Fat 10g| Carbs 15g| Protein 35g

Rib Eye With Chimichurri Sauce

Prep time: 15 minutes | Cook time:15 minutes | Serves 4

FOR THE CHIMICHURRI

- ½ cup good-quality olive oil
- ½ cup finely chopped fresh parsley
- 2 tablespoons red wine vinegar
- 2 tablespoons finely chopped fresh cilantro
- 1½ tablespoons minced garlic
- 1 tablespoon finely chopped chile pepper
- ½ teaspoon sea salt
- ¼ teaspoon freshly ground black pepper
- For The Steak
- 4 (5-ounce) rib eye steaks
- 1 tablespoon good-quality olive oil
- Sea salt, for seasoning
- Freshly ground black pepper, for seasoning

TO MAKE THE CHIMICHURRI

1. Make the chimichurri. In a medium bowl, stir together the olive oil, parsley, vinegar, cilantro, garlic, chile, salt, and pepper. Let it stand for 15 minutes to mellow the flavors.

TO MAKE THE STEAK

1. Prepare the steaks. Let the steaks come to room temperature and lightly oil them with the olive oil and season them with salt and pepper.
2. Grill the steaks. Preheat the grill to high heat. Grill the steaks for 6 to 7 minutes per side for medium (140°F internal temperature) or until they're done the way you like them.
3. Rest and serve. Let the steaks rest for 10 minutes and then serve them topped with generous spoonfuls of the chimichurri sauce.

PER SERVING

Calories: 503 | Total Fat: 42g | Total Carbs: 1g | Fiber: 0g | Net Carbs: 1g | Sodium: 385mg | Protein: 29g

Cheesy Beef Stroganoff Casserole

Prep time: 8 minutes | Cook time: 47 minutes | Serves 8

- 2 pounds stew beef, cut into bite-sized pieces
- 1½ teaspoons kosher salt
- ½ teaspoon ground black pepper
- 3 tablespoons butter, divided
- 2 cups sliced white mushrooms
- ½ cup sliced yellow onions
- 1 tablespoon minced garlic
- 1 cup beef broth, store-bought or homemade
- 1 teaspoon Worcestershire sauce
- ¾ cup full-fat sour cream
- ¼ teaspoon xanthan gum
- ½ teaspoon fresh thyme leaves
- 1 batch Cheesy Cauliflower Puree
- 2 tablespoons chopped fresh parsley, for garnish (optional)

1. Season the beef with the salt and pepper. Melt 2 tablespoons of the butter in a large sauté pan over high heat. Add the beef and sear for 3 minutes, or until browned, stirring occasionally. Remove the beef to a bowl and set aside.
2. Lower the heat to medium. Add the mushrooms to the pan and cook until golden brown, about 5 minutes. Remove to the bowl with the beef. Add the onions, garlic, and remaining tablespoon of butter to the pan. Cook until the onions are translucent, about 4 minutes. Remove to the bowl with the beef and mushrooms.
3. Add the beef broth and Worcestershire sauce to the pan and whisk up all of the browned bits into the liquid. Whisk in the sour cream and xanthan gum and cook over medium heat until reduced and thickened, about 5 minutes.
4. Add the beef, mushroom, and onion mixture back to the pan and stir to coat. Remove from the heat and stir in the thyme. Taste and season with more salt and pepper, if desired.
5. Preheat the oven to 375°F. Transfer the beef mixture to a 2-quart or 9-inch square casserole dish. Spread the cauliflower puree evenly over the top of the beef mixture. Bake for 30 minutes, or until the top is turning golden and the stroganoff is bubbling at the edges.
6. Remove the casserole from the oven and let cool for 5 minutes. Garnish with fresh parsley, if desired, and serve hot.

PER SERVING

Calories: 518 | Fat: 41g | Protein: 27g | Carbs: 10.5g | Fiber: 4g | Net Carbs: 6.5g

T-Bone Steak With Citrus Marinade

Prep time: 5 minutes | Cook time:15 minutes | Serves 4

- ¼ cup good-quality olive oil
- ¼ cup freshly squeezed lime juice
- 2 tablespoons balsamic vinegar
- 2 tablespoons freshly squeezed orange juice
- 1 tablespoon minced garlic
- 1 tablespoon finely chopped fresh basil
- 4 T-bone steaks (about 1½ pounds total)

1. Marinate the beef. In a medium bowl, stir together the olive oil, lime juice, vinegar, orange juice, garlic, and basil. Pour the marinade into a resealable plastic bag and add the steaks to the bag. Squeeze out the excess air and seal the bag. Refrigerate the steak to marinate for 30 minutes.
2. Grill the steak. Preheat the grill to medium-high heat. Remove the steak from the marinade and grill it for 6 to 7 minutes per side for medium (140°F internal temperature) or until it's done the way you like it. Throw out any leftover marinade.
3. Rest and serve. Let the steak rest for 10 minutes. Divide the steaks between four plates and serve them immediately.

PER SERVING

Calories: 524 | Total Fat: 42g | Total Carbs: 3g | Fiber: 0g | Net Carbs: 3g | Sodium: 91mg | Protein: 32g

Sunday Pork Tacos

Prep time: 5 minutes | Cook time:8 hours 10 minutes| Serves 4

- 3 lb pork shoulder
- 2 cups chicken broth
- Juice of 1 orange
- 1 small onion, chopped
- 4 coconut taco shells
- Sea salt and pepper to taste
- 1 tsp ground cumin
- 1 tsp garlic powder
- ½ tsp dried coriander

1. Rub the pork with salt, cumin, garlic powder, coriander, and pepper.
2. Put it in your slow cooker.
3. Pour the broth and orange juice around the pork.
4. Scatter the onion around the pork.
5. Cover the cooker and set on "Low".
6. Cook for 8 hours.
7. Transfer the pork to a work surface and shred it with a fork.
8. Serve in taco shells and enjoy!

PER SERVING

Cal 1150| Fat 85g| Carbs 12g| Protein 82g

Beef Sausage Meat Loaf

Prep time: 10 minutes | Cook time:1 Hour, 15 minutes | Serves 6

- 1½ pounds Italian sausage meat
- 1 pound grass-fed ground beef
- ½ cup almond flour
- 1 egg, lightly beaten
- ½ onion, finely chopped
- ½ red bell pepper, chopped
- 2 teaspoons minced garlic
- 1 teaspoon dried oregano
- ¼ teaspoon sea salt
- ⅛ teaspoon freshly ground black pepper

1. Preheat the oven. Set the oven temperature to 400°F.
2. Make the meat loaf. In a large bowl, mix together the sausage, ground beef, almond flour, cream, egg, onion, red bell pepper, garlic, oregano, salt, and pepper until everything is well combined. Press the mixture into a 9-inch loaf pan.
3. Bake. Bake for 1 hour to 1 hour and 15 minutes, or until the meat loaf is cooked through. Drain off and throw out any grease and let the meat loaf stand for 10 minutes.
4. Serve. Cut the meat loaf into six slices, divide them between six plates, and serve it immediately.

PER SERVING

Calories: 394 | Total Fat: 34g | Total Carbs: 1g | Fiber: 0g | Net Carbs: 1g | Sodium: 325mg | Protein: 19g

Juicy No-Fail Burger

Prep time: 10 minutes | Cook time:15 minutes | Serves 4

- 1 pound grass-fed ground beef
- 1 egg, lightly beaten
- ½ onion, finely chopped
- 1 teaspoon minced garlic
- 1 teaspoon Worcestershire sauce
- ¼ teaspoon sea salt
- ⅛ teaspoon freshly ground black pepper
- 1 tablespoon olive oil

1. Make the burgers. In a medium bowl, combine the ground beef, egg, onion, garlic, Worcestershire sauce, parsley, salt, and pepper until everything is well mixed. Form the mixture into four equal patties, each about ¾ inch thick. Lightly oil the patties with olive oil.
2. Grill the burgers. Preheat the grill to medium heat. Grill the burgers, turning them once, until they're just cooked through (160°F internal temperature), about 8 minutes per side.
3. Serve. Let the burgers rest for 5 minutes, then serve them immediately.

PER SERVING

Calories: 379 | Total Fat: 33g | Total Carbs: 1g | Fiber: 0g | Net Carbs: 1g | Sodium: 238mg | Protein: 19g

Coffee-Rubbed Rib-Eyes with Balsamic Butter

Prep time: 5 minutes | Cook time: 15 minutes | Serves 2

FOR THE RUB:

- 1 tablespoon ground coffee
- 1 tablespoon unsweetened cocoa powder
- 2 teaspoons kosher salt
- ¼ teaspoon cayenne pepper
- 2 (8-ounce) bone-in rib-eye steaks, room temperature
- For The Balsamic Butter:
- 3 tablespoons butter, softened
- 2 tablespoons balsamic vinegar (no sugar added)
- 1 teaspoon granulated erythritol
- For garnish (optional):
- Chopped fresh parsley

1. Preheat a grill to medium heat. Combine the coffee, cocoa powder, salt, and cayenne in a small bowl. Rub the steaks generously with the coffee mixture.
2. Grill the steaks on direct heat for 6 minutes (for medium) to 8 minutes (for medium-well) per side, or until your desired doneness is reached.
3. Remove the steaks from the grill and let rest for 5 minutes. Meanwhile, place the butter, balsamic vinegar, and sweetener in a small bowl and mix with a fork until blended. Serve the steaks with a generous dollop of balsamic butter. Garnish with chopped parsley, if desired.

PER SERVING

Calories: 583 | Fat: 45g | Protein: 53g | Carbs: 4g | Fiber: 1g | Erythritol: 2g | Net Carbs: 3g

Spicy Lime Pork Tenderloins

Prep time: 5 minutes | Cook time: 7 hours 10 minutes | Serves 4

- 2 lb pork tenderloins
- 1 cup chicken broth
- ¼ cup lime juice
- 3 tsp chili powder
- 2 tsp garlic powder
- 1 tsp ginger powder
- ½ tsp sea salt

1. Combine chili powder, garlic powder, ginger powder, and salt in a bowl.
2. Rub the pork all over with the spice mixture and put it in your slow cooker.
3. Pour in the broth and lime juice around the pork.
4. Cover with the lid and cook for 7 hours on "Low".
5. Remove the pork from the slow cooker and let rest for 5 minutes.
6. Slice the pork against the grain into medallions before serving.

PER SERVING

Cal 260| Fat 6g| Carbs 5g| Protein 49g

Pizza With Prosciutto, Ricotta, And Truffle Oil

Prep time: 15 minutes | Cook time: 7 minutes | Serves 4

- For The Pizza Crust
- 1¾ cups shredded mozzarella cheese
- 3 tablespoons plain cream cheese
- 1 cup almond flour
- ½ teaspoon dried basil
- ½ teaspoon dried oregano
- Pinch sea salt
- 1 egg, lightly beaten
- Olive oil cooking spray
- For The Pizza
- 6 ounces prosciutto
- 8 ounces ricotta cheese
- Truffle oil

TO MAKE THE PIZZA CRUST

1. Preheat the oven. Set the oven temperature to broil.
2. Melt the cheeses. Stir together the mozzarella and cream cheese in a large microwave-safe bowl and microwave on high for 1 minute. Stir the cheeses and heat them again for 30 seconds to 1 minute until they're completely melted.
3. Add the dry ingredients. Stir in the almond flour, basil, oregano, and salt until everything is well mixed and set it aside to cool to room temperature, about 10 minutes.
4. Finish the dough. When the mixture has cooled enough that it won't cook the egg, mix in the egg until it's well blended, then gather the dough into a ball.
5. Roll the dough. Lay a piece of parchment paper on a baking sheet and spray it lightly with olive oil. Place the dough on the sheet in the center and press it down with your fingers to form a disc until it is about ⅓ inch thick. It's fine if the dough looks rustic and not perfectly round.
6. Broil the dough. Broil the dough until it is golden and firm, about 4 minutes.

TO MAKE THE PIZZA

1. Preheat the oven. Preheat the oven to 425°F.
2. Top the pizza. Place the prosciutto over the pizza crust. Then use a small ice cream scoop to distribute about 6 scoops of ricotta cheese on top, evenly spacing the cheese mounds. Do not spread it out because the cheese will melt when baked. Drizzle the truffle oil with a spoon all over the pizza.
3. Bake the pizza. Place the pizza back in the oven and bake until the ricotta is melted, about 5 to 7 minutes.
4. Serve. Cut it into slices, and serve it immediately.

PER SERVING

Calories: 446 | Total Fat: 31g | Total Carbs: 10g | Fiber: 2g | Net Carbs: 8g | Sodium: 985mg | Protein: 32g

Flaky Beef Empanadas

Prep time: 30 minutes | Cook time:25 minutes | Serves 6

- For The Dough
- 1 cup mozzarella cheese, shredded
- 5 tablespoons cream cheese
- ¾ cup almond flour
- 2 tablespoons coconut milk
- 1 tablespoon coconut flour
- 1 egg, lightly beaten
- 1 teaspoon garlic powder
- ½ teaspoon sea salt
- For The Filling
- ¼ cup grass-fed butter
- 1 pound grass-fed ground beef
- 1 onion, chopped
- 1 tablespoon minced garlic
- 2 tablespoons sugar-free tomato paste
- 2 teaspoons ground cumin
- 2 teaspoons dried oregano
- 1 teaspoon chili powder
- Sea salt, for seasoning
- Freshly ground black pepper, for seasoning

TO MAKE THE DOUGH

1. Melt the cheeses. In a small saucepan over low heat, melt the mozzarella and cream cheese together, stirring often. Remove the pan from the heat.
2. Mix the dough. Transfer the cheese mixture to a medium bowl and stir in the almond flour, coconut milk, coconut flour, egg, garlic powder, and salt until everything is well blended and the mixture holds together in a ball. Cover the bowl with plastic wrap, pressing it down onto the surface of the dough, and place the bowl in the refrigerator for 30 minutes.

TO MAKE THE FILLING

1. Cook the beef. In a large skillet over medium-high heat, melt the butter. Add the beef and cook it until it's browned, about 7 minutes.
2. Finish the filling. Add the onion and garlic and sauté until they've softened, about 4 minutes. Stir in the tomato paste, cumin, oregano, and chili powder. Season the filling with salt and pepper and set it aside to cool.

TO MAKE THE EMPANADAS

1. Preheat the oven. Set the oven temperature to 425°F. Line a baking sheet with parchment paper.
2. Cut the dough. Spread some parchment paper on your work surface. Press the dough out into a thin layer on the paper, then cut the dough into 12 (3-inch) circles.
3. Fill the dough. Spoon the filling equally onto the middle of each dough circle. Fold the dough over and press the edges together using a fork to seal them.
4. Bake. Transfer the empanadas to the baking sheet and bake them for 10 to 12 minutes until they're golden brown.
5. Serve. Divide the empanadas between six plates and serve them immediately.

PER SERVING

Calories: 436 | Total Fat: 38g | Total Carbs: 4g | Fiber: 1g | Net Carbs: 3g | Sodium: 229mg | Protein: 19g

Simple Liver And Onions

Prep time: 10 minutes | Cook time:25 minutes | Serves 4

- ½ cup grass-fed butter
- ¼ cup extra-virgin olive oil
- 2 onions, thinly sliced
- ½ cup white wine
- 1 pound calf's liver, trimmed and cut into strips
- 1 tablespoon balsamic vinegar
- 2 tablespoons chopped fresh parsley
- Sea salt, for seasoning
- Freshly ground black pepper, for seasoning

1. Sauté the onions. In a large skillet over medium heat, warm the butter and olive oil. Add the onions to the skillet and sauté them until they've softened, about 5 minutes. Stir in the white wine and reduce the heat to medium-low. Cover the skillet and cook, stirring frequently, until the onions are very soft and lightly browned, about 15 minutes. Transfer the onions with a slotted spoon to a plate.
2. Cook the liver. Increase the heat to high and stir in the liver strips and the vinegar. Sauté the liver until it's done the way you like it, about 4 minutes for medium rare.
3. Finish the dish. Return the onions to the skillet along with the parsley, stirring to combine them. Season the liver and onions with salt and pepper.
4. Serve. Divide the liver and onions between four plates and serve immediately.

PER SERVING

Calories: 497 | Total Fat: 40g | Total Carbs: 8g | Fiber: 3g | Net Carbs: 5g | Sodium: 103mg | Protein: 23g

Tomato & Lentil Lamb Ragù
Prep time: 5 minutes | Cook time: 35 minutes | Serves 4

- 1 red onion, chopped
- 4 garlic cloves, minced
- 1 lb ground lamb
- 14 oz canned diced tomatoes
- 1 cup chicken broth
- 2 tbsp extra-virgin olive oil
- ½ cup green lentils
- Sea salt and pepper to taste
- 1 tsp ginger powder
- 1 tsp ground cumin

1. Warm the olive oil in a large pan over high heat.
2. Add the onion and garlic sauté for 3 minutes.
3. Add the ground lamb, breaking it up with a spoon.
4. Brown for 3-4 minutes.
5. Stir in the tomatoes, chicken broth, lentils, salt, ginger powder, cumin, and pepper.
6. Simmer for 20 minutes, or until the lentils are cooked and most of the liquid has evaporated.
7. Serve and enjoy!

PER SERVING

Cal 400| Fat 15g| Carbs 23g| Protein 40g

Port Wine Garlicky Lamb
Prep time: 5 minutes | Cook time: 25 minutes | Serves 4

- 2 lb lamb shanks
- 1 tbsp olive oil
- ½ cup Port wine
- 1 tbsp tomato paste
- 10 peeled whole garlic cloves
- ½ cup chicken broth
- 1 tsp balsamic vinegar
- ½ tsp dried rosemary
- 1 tbsp olive oil

1. Heat the oil in the Instant Pot on "Sauté" and brown the lamb shanks on all sides.
2. Add the garlic and cook until lightly browned, no more than 2 minutes.
3. Stir in the rest of the ingredients, except the oil and vinegar.
4. Seal the lid and cook for 20 minutes on "Manual" on high.
5. When cooking is complete, release the pressure naturally for 10 minutes.
6. Remove the lamb shanks and let the sauce boil for 5 minutes with the lid off.
7. Stir in the vinegar and butter.
8. Serve the gravy poured over the shanks.

PER SERVING

Cal 620| Fat 35g| Carbs 9g| Protein 60g

Beef Burrito Bowl
Prep time: 5 minutes | Cook time: 15 minutes | Serves 1

- ½ cup Basic Cauliflower Rice, hot
- 2/3 cup Easy No-Chop Chili, hot
- ½ cup shredded romaine lettuce
- ¼ cup shredded cheddar cheese
- ¼ cup Easy Keto Guacamole
- ¼ cup Restaurant-Style Salsa
- ¼ cup full-fat sour cream
- 1 tablespoon chopped fresh cilantro, for garnish (optional)

1. Arrange all of the ingredients in a serving bowl as shown, or place the cauliflower rice in the bowl first, then top the cauliflower rice with the remaining ingredients. Garnish with the cilantro, if desired. Serve immediately.

PER SERVING

Calories: 441 | Fat: 26g | Protein: 43g | Carbs: 10g | Fiber: 3g | Net Carbs: 7g

Lettuce-Wrapped Beef Roast
Prep time: 5 minutes | Cook time: 8 hours 10 minutes | Serves 4

- 2 lb beef chuck roast
- 1 shallot, diced
- 1 cup beef broth
- 3 tbsp coconut aminos
- 1 tbsp rice vinegar
- 1 tsp garlic powder
- 1 tsp olive oil
- ½ tsp ground ginger
- ¼ tsp red pepper flakes
- 8 romaine lettuce leaves
- 1 tbsp sesame seeds
- 1 scallion, diced

1. Place the beef, shallot, broth, coconut aminos, vinegar, garlic powder, olive oil, ginger, and red pepper flakes in your slow cooker.
2. Cover the cooker and set to "Low".
3. Cook for 8 hours.
4. Scoop spoonfuls of the beef mixture into each lettuce leaf.
5. Top with sesame seeds and scallion.

PER SERVING

Cal 425| Fat 22g| Carbs 12g| Protein 45g

Korean BBQ Beef Wraps

Prep time: 8 minutes, plus 2 hours to marinate | Cook time: 8 minutes | Serves 4

FOR THE BBQ BEEF:

- 1 pound boneless beef sirloin, thinly sliced
- ¼ cup chopped scallions
- 2 tablespoons granulated erythritol
- 2 tablespoons peeled and minced fresh ginger
- 1 tablespoon minced garlic
- 2 teaspoons cayenne pepper
- ¼ cup filtered water
- ¼ cup wheat-free soy sauce
- 1 tablespoon toasted sesame oil
- For Serving:
- 8 large red or green lettuce leaves
- 1 cup Basic Cauliflower Rice
- For garnish (optional):
- Sliced scallions
- Thinly sliced red chili peppers

1. Place the beef, scallions, sweetener, ginger, garlic, cayenne pepper, water, soy sauce, and sesame oil in a medium-sized bowl and stir well to coat. Cover and place in the refrigerator to marinate for 2 hours or overnight.
2. Heat a large skillet over medium-high heat. Add the beef (reserve the marinade) to the skillet and cook for about 3 minutes, or until just cooked through. Remove the meat from the pan and set aside.
3. Return the skillet to the stove and pour the marinade into it. Bring to a boil and simmer for 2 minutes; if you want to thin out the sauce, add 1 or 2 tablespoons of filtered water.
4. Add the cooked meat back to the sauce and stir to coat. To serve each portion, place 2 lettuce leaves on a plate, then add ¼ cup of the cauliflower rice and one-quarter of the BBQ beef. Top with sliced scallions and chili peppers, if desired. Repeat for the remaining servings.

PER SERVING

Calories: 287 | Fat: 18g | Protein: 26g | Carbs: 5g | Fiber: 1.5g | Erythritol: 6g | Net Carbs: 3.5g

Meatballs alla Parmigiana

Prep time: 10 minutes | Cook time: 40 minutes | Serves 4

- 1 pound ground beef (80/20)
- 2 tablespoons chopped fresh parsley, plus more for garnish if desired
- ⅓ cup grated Parmesan cheese
- ¼ cup superfine blanched almond flour
- 1 large egg, beaten
- 1 teaspoon kosher salt
- ¼ teaspoon onion powder
- ¼ teaspoon dried oregano leaves
- ¼ cup warm filtered water
- 1 cup marinara sauce, store-bought or homemade
- 1 cup shredded whole-milk mozzarella cheese

1. Preheat the oven to 350°F. Line a 15 by 10-inch sheet pan with foil or parchment paper.
2. Put the ground beef, parsley, Parmesan, almond flour, egg, salt, pepper, garlic powder, onion powder, oregano, and water in a medium-sized bowl. Mix thoroughly by hand until fully combined.
3. Form the meat mixture into 12 meatballs about 2 inches in diameter and place them 2 inches apart on the sheet pan. Bake for 20 minutes.
4. Place the meatballs in a casserole dish large enough to fit all of the meatballs. Spoon the marinara evenly over the meatballs, then sprinkle the cheese over the meatballs. Bake for 20 minutes, or until the meatballs are cooked through, the sauce is bubbling, and the cheese is golden. Garnish with chopped fresh parsley, if desired.

PER SERVING

Calories: 430 | Fat: 31g | Protein: 33g | Carbs: 5g | Fiber: 2g | Net Carbs: 3g

Smoky Lamb Souvlaki

Prep time: 5 minutes | Cook time:20 minutes | Serves 4

- 1 lb lamb shoulder, cubed
- 2 tbsp olive oil
- 1 tbsp apple cider vinegar
- 2 tsp crushed fennel seeds
- 2 tsp smoked paprika
- Salt and garlic powder to taste

1. Blend the olive oil, cider vinegar, crushed fennel seeds, smoked paprika, garlic powder, and sea salt in a large bowl.
2. Stir in the lamb.
3. Cover the bowl and refrigerate it for 1 hour to marinate.
4. Preheat a frying pan over high heat.
5. Thread 4-5 pieces of lamb each onto 8 skewers.
6. Fry for 3-4 minutes per side until cooked through.
7. Serve.

PER SERVING

Cal 275| Fat 15g| Carbs 1g| Protein 31g

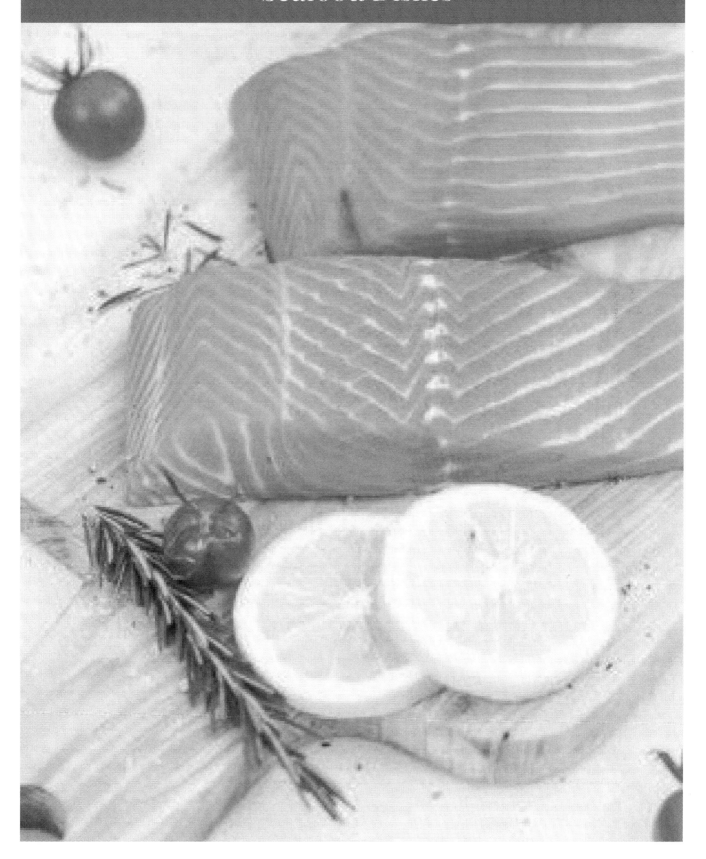

Chapter 8
Seafood Dishes

Spicy Shrimp Scampi

Prep time: 5 minutes | Cook time:20 minutes | Serves 4

- 1 ½ lb shrimp, peeled and tails removed
- 1 tsp ancho chili powder
- ¼ cup coconut oil
- 1 tsp paprika
- 1 onion, finely chopped
- 1 red bell pepper, chopped
- 2 garlic cloves, minced
- 1 lemon, zested and juiced
- Sea salt and pepper to taste

1. Warm the coconut oil in a skillet over medium heat.
2. Add the onion and red bell pepper and cook for 6 minutes until tender.
3. Put in shrimp and cook for 5 minutes until it's pink.
4. Mix in garlic and cook for another 30 seconds.
5. Add lemon juice, lemon zest, ancho chili powder, paprika, salt, and pepper and simmer for 3 minutes.
6. Serve warm.

PER SERVING

Cal 350| Fat 17g| Carbs 11g| Protein 1g

Creamy Crabmeat

Prep time: 5 minutes | Cook time:10 minutes | Serves 4

- ¼ cup olive oil
- 1 small red onion, chopped
- 1 lb lump crabmeat
- ½ celery stalk, chopped
- ½ cup plain yogurt
- ¼ cup chicken broth

1. Season the crabmeat with some salt and pepper.
2. Heat the oil in your Instant Pot on "Sauté".
3. Add celery and onion and cook for 3 minutes, or until soft.
4. Add the crabmeat and stir in the broth.
5. Seal and lock the lid and set to "Steam" for 5 minutes on high pressure.
6. Once the cooking is complete, do a quick release and carefully open the lid.
7. Stir in the yogurt and serve.

PER SERVING

Cal 450| Fat 10g| Carbs 12g| Protein 40g

Yummy Fish Curry

Prep time: 5 minutes | Cook time: 25 minutes | Serves 4

- 2 shallots, chopped
- 2 garlic cloves, minced
- 2 tbsp coconut oil
- 1 tbsp minced fresh ginger
- 2 tsp curry powder
- 2 cups cubed butternut squash
- 2 cups chopped broccoli
- 1 cup vegetable broth
- 1 lb firm white fish fillets
- ¼ cup chopped cilantro
- 1 scallion, sliced thin
- Lemon wedges, for garnish

1. Melt the coconut oil in a large pot over medium heat.
2. Add the shallots, garlic, ginger, curry powder, salt, and pepper.
3. Sauté for 5 minutes.
4. Add the butternut squash and broccoli.
5. Sauté for 2 minutes more.
6. Stir in the coconut milk and vegetable broth and bring to a boil.
7. Reduce the heat to simmer and add the fish.
8. Cover the pot and simmer for 5 minutes, or until the fish is cooked through.
9. Remove and discard the lemongrass.
10. Ladle the curry into a serving bowl.
11. Garnish with the cilantro and scallion and serve with lemon wedges.

PER SERVING

Cal 550| Fat 39g| Carbs 22g| Protein 33g

Lime-Avocado Ahi Poke

Prep time: 5 minutes | Cook time:5 minutes | Serves 4

- 1 lb sushi-grade ahi tuna, cubed
- 1 cucumber, sliced
- 1 large avocado, diced
- 3 tbsp coconut aminos
- 3 scallions, thinly sliced
- 1 serrano chile, minced
- 1 tsp lime juice
- 1 tsp toasted sesame seeds
- ¼ tsp ground ginger

1. Mix the ahi tuna cubes with the coconut aminos, scallions, serrano chile, olive oil, lime juice, sesame seeds, and ginger in a large bowl.
2. Cover the bowl with plastic wrap and marinate in the fridge for 15 minutes.
3. Add the diced avocado to the bowl of ahi poke and stir to incorporate.
4. Arrange the cucumber rounds on a serving plate.
5. Spoon the ahi poke over the cucumber and serve.

PER SERVING

Cal 210| Fat 15g| Carbs 10g| Protein 9g

Crab Tacos

Prep time: 5 minutes | Cook time: 5 minutes | Serves 4

- 1 cup (230 g) cooked crab leg meat
- 2 small tomatoes, diced
- ⅓ cup (55 g) diced radishes
- Juice of 1 lime
- 3 tablespoons extra-virgin olive oil
- 3 tablespoons finely chopped green bell pepper
- 2 tablespoons finely chopped yellow bell pepper
- 2 tablespoons finely chopped fresh cilantro, plus more for garnish
- 2 tablespoons Sriracha sauce
- 1 tablespoon finely chopped fresh mint
- ¼ teaspoon finely ground gray sea salt
- 8 Bendy Tortillas (here), for serving

1. Place all the ingredients except the tortillas in a large bowl. Toss to combine.
2. Divide the crab mixture evenly among the 8 tortillas. Garnish with additional cilantro, if using, and serve.

PER 2 TACOS

Calories: 297 | Calories From Fat: 176 | Total Fat: 19.5g | Saturated Fat: 4.4g | Cholesterol: 129mg Sodium: 747mg | Carbs: 5.5g | Dietary Fiber: 1.1g | Net Carbs: 4.4g | Sugars: 3.4g | Protein: 24.9g

Stuffed Trout

Prep time: 5 minutes | Cook time: 20 minutes | Serves 4

- 2 (7-ounce/200-g) head-off, gutted trout
- 2 tablespoons refined avocado oil or melted coconut oil
- 2 teaspoons dried dill weed
- 1 teaspoon dried thyme leaves
- ½ teaspoon ground black pepper
- ¼ teaspoon finely ground gray sea salt
- ½ lemon, sliced
- 1 green onion, green part only, sliced in half lengthwise

1. Preheat the oven to 400°F (205°C).
2. Place the fish in a large cast-iron frying pan or on an unlined rimmed baking sheet and coat with the oil. In a small bowl, mix together the dried herbs, pepper, and salt. Sprinkle the fish—top, bottom, and inside—with the herb mixture.
3. Open up the fish and place the lemon and green onion slices inside. Lay it flat on the pan or baking sheet and transfer to the oven. Bake for up to 20 minutes, until the desired doneness is reached.
4. Cut the fish in half before transferring to a serving platter.

PER SERVING

Calories: 219 | Calories From Fat: 108 | Total Fat: 12g | Saturated Fat: 2g | Cholesterol: 74mg Sodium: 186mg | Carbs: 0.9g | Dietary Fiber: 0g | Net Carbs: 0.9g | Sugars: 0g | Protein: 26.9g

Crispy Salmon Steaks With Sweet Cabbage

Prep time: 10 minutes | Cook time: 40 minutes | Serves 4

SWEET CABBAGE

- ¼ cup (60 ml) refined avocado oil or macadamia nut oil
- ⅓ cup (55 g) sliced red onions
- 4 cups (470 g) sliced red cabbage
- ⅓ cup (80 ml) red wine, such as Pinot Noir, Merlot, or Cabernet Sauvignon
- ¼ cup (60 ml) chicken bone broth
- 1 tablespoon balsamic vinegar
- ½ teaspoon finely ground gray sea salt
- ¼ teaspoon ground black pepper

SALMON

- 4 salmon steaks (6 ounces/170 g each)
- 3 tablespoons refined avocado oil or macadamia nut oil
- Finely ground gray sea salt and ground black pepper
- 2 tablespoons chopped fresh parsley, for garnish

1. Prepare the cabbage: Place ¼ cup (60 ml) of avocado oil and the red onions in a large frying pan over medium heat. Sauté the onions for 5 minutes. Add the sliced cabbage and continue to cook for 5 minutes, or until lightly wilted. Add the wine, bone broth, vinegar, salt, and pepper. Cover, reduce the heat to medium-low, and cook for 25 minutes. During the last 5 minutes of cooking, remove the lid and continue to cook, uncovered, to allow some of the juices to evaporate.
2. Meanwhile, place an oven rack in the top position and set the broiler to low. (If your oven doesn't have a low broil setting, just "broil" is fine.)
3. Place the salmon steaks on an unlined rimmed baking sheet or in a large cast-iron frying pan. Drizzle with 3 tablespoons of avocado oil and sprinkle with salt and pepper. For medium-done steaks, still slightly translucent in the center, broil for 9 minutes; for fully cooked steaks, opaque throughout, broil for 12 minutes.
4. Divide the cabbage among 4 plates, top each plate with a salmon steak, and serve garnished with parsley.

PER SERVING

Calories: 485 | Calories From Fat: 310 | Total Fat: 34.5g | Saturated Fat: 4.6g | Cholesterol: 75mg Sodium: 499mg | Carbs: 8.3g | Dietary Fiber: 3.3g | Net Carbs: 5g | Sugars: 4.4g | Protein: 35.2g

Prosciutto-Wrapped Fish Fillets With Mediterranean Vegetables

Prep time: 15 minutes | Cook time: 30 minutes | Serves 6

VEGETABLES

- 10½ ounces (300 g) endive or radicchio, roughly chopped
- 6 canned artichoke hearts
- ½ cup (70 g) raw pecan halves
- ⅓ cup (80 ml) refined avocado oil or melted lard
- 4 green onions, green parts only, chopped
- Juice of 1 lime
- 1 (1-in/2.5-cm) piece fresh ginger root, grated
- Leaves from 1 sprig fresh tarragon
- ½ teaspoon finely ground gray sea salt
- ¼ teaspoon ground black pepper

FISH

- 1 pound (455 g) trout, tilapia, or catfish fillets
- Finely ground gray sea salt and ground black pepper
- 9 ounces (255 g) thinly sliced prosciutto

FOR GARNISH (OPTIONAL)

- Fresh parsley leaves
- Lime wedges

1. Preheat the oven to 350°F (177°C).
2. In a large bowl, place the ingredients for the vegetables. Toss to coat before transferring to a shallow 1½-quart (1.4-L) casserole dish.
3. Place the fish fillets on a clean surface. Sprinkle with salt and pepper. One at a time, wrap each fillet with 2 or 3 pieces of prosciutto. Once wrapped, place on top of the endive mixture.
4. Bake for 30 minutes, or until the sides of the casserole start to brown and the fish flakes with a fork.
5. Divide the fish and vegetables among 6 plates and garnish with fresh parsley and lime wedges, if desired. Serve!

PER SERVING

Calories: 436 | Calories From Fat: 265 | Total Fat: 29.5g | Saturated Fat: 4.4g | Cholesterol: 78mg Sodium: 772mg | Carbs: 10g | Dietary Fiber: 5.5g | Net Carbs: 4.5g | Sugars: 1.3g | Protein: 32.6g

Baked Mahi Mahi in Garlic Parsley Butter

Prep time: 5 minutes | Cook time: 15 minutes | Serves 4

- 3 tablespoons butter, melted
- 2 tablespoons chopped fresh parsley
- 1 tablespoon grated lemon zest
- 1 tablespoon lemon juice
- ½ teaspoon kosher salt
- ½ teaspoon minced garlic
- 1 (1-pound) mahi mahi (or other firm white fish) fillet, cut into 4 pieces
- ¼ cup Keto Breadcrumbs

1. Preheat the oven to 350°F.
2. Place the melted butter, parsley, lemon zest, lemon juice, salt, and garlic in a small bowl and mix well.
3. Place the fish fillets in a small casserole dish. Pour the butter mixture over the fillets. Top the fillets with the keto breadcrumbs. Bake for 15 minutes, or until the fish is flaky and opaque in the center and the tops are golden brown.
4. Remove the fillets from the oven and serve immediately.

PER SERVING

Calories: 254 | Fat: 23g | Protein: 23g | Carbs: 2g | Fiber: 1g | Net Carbs: 1g

Trout Fillets with Almond Crust

Prep time: 5 minutes | Cook time:15 minutes | Serves 4

- ½ cup whole-wheat breadcrumbs
- 2 trout fillets
- 1 tbsp extra-virgin olive oil
- 1 tsp Italian seasoning
- 1 lemon, juiced and zested
- ½ cup chopped almonds

1. Preheat your oven to 375°F.
2. Mix breadcrumbs, Italian seasoning, lemon zest, lemon juice, and half of the almonds in a shallow dish.
3. Lay the fillets skin side down onto the oiled baking tray and then flip over so that both sides of your fish are coated in the oil.
4. Roll the fillets into the nut mixture on both sides to coat.
5. Return to the baking tray.
6. Bake for 6-7 minutes on each side and serve.

PER SERVING

Cal 870| Fat 50g| Carbs 56g| Protein 51g

Salmon Cakes With Dill Cream Sauce

Prep time: 5 minutes | Cook time: 15 minutes | Serves 4

- ¼ cup (60 ml) refined avocado oil or macadamia nut oil, for the pan

SALMON CAKES

- 2 (7½-ounce/213-g) cans salmon, drained
- 2 large eggs
- 2 tablespoons roughly chopped fresh dill
- Juice of ½ lemon
- ½ teaspoon finely ground gray sea salt

DILL CREAM SAUCE

- 1 cup (240 ml) coconut cream
- Juice of ½ lemon
- 2 teaspoons finely chopped fresh dill
- ½ teaspoon ground black pepper

1. Warm the oil in a large frying pan over medium heat for 2 minutes.
2. Meanwhile, make the salmon cakes: Place the salmon, eggs, dill, lemon juice, and salt in a high-powered blender or food processor and blend until smooth. Spoon about 3 tablespoons of the mixture into your palm, roll it into a ball, and flatten it like a burger patty. Repeat with the remaining salmon mixture, making a total of 8 patties.
3. Pan-fry the cakes in the hot oil for 3 to 5 minutes on the first side, then turn them over and fry for 3 minutes on the second side, just until lightly golden. Transfer to a cooling rack. You may have to fry the cakes in batches if your pan isn't large enough to fit them without overcrowding.
4. Meanwhile, prepare the dill cream sauce: Place all the sauce ingredients in a medium-sized bowl and stir to combine.
5. Divide the fried cakes among 4 plates, drizzle with the cream sauce, and dig in!

PER 2 CAKES AND ¼ CUP/60 ML SAUCE

Calories: 459 | Calories From Fat: 337 | Total Fat: 37.4g | Saturated Fat: 16.4g | Cholesterol: 140mg Sodium: 331mg | Carbs: 4.7g | Dietary Fiber: 1.6g | Net Carbs: 3.1g | Sugars: 2.5g | Protein: 25.8g

Sardine Fritter Wraps

Prep time: 5 minutes | Cook time: 8 minutes | Serves 4

- ⅓ cup (80 ml) refined avocado oil, for frying

FRITTERS

- 2 (4.375-ounce/125-g) cans sardines, drained
- ½ cup (55 g) blanched almond flour
- 2 large eggs
- 2 tablespoons finely chopped fresh parsley
- 2 tablespoons finely diced red bell pepper
- 2 cloves garlic, minced
- ½ teaspoon finely ground gray sea salt
- ¼ teaspoon ground black pepper

FOR SERVING

- 8 romaine lettuce leaves
- 1 small English cucumber, sliced thin
- 8 tablespoons (105 g) mayonnaise, homemade (here) or store-bought
- Thinly sliced green onions

1. Pour the avocado oil into a large frying pan. Heat on medium for a couple of minutes.
2. Meanwhile, prepare the fritters: Place the fritter ingredients in a medium-sized bowl and stir to combine, being careful not to mash the heck out of the sardines. Spoon about 1 tablespoon of the mixture into the palm of your hand and roll it into a ball, then flatten it like a burger patty. Repeat with the remaining fritter mixture, making a total of 16 small patties.
3. Fry the fritters in the hot oil for 2 minutes per side, then transfer to a cooling rack. You may have to fry the fritters in batches if your pan isn't large enough to fit them all without overcrowding.
4. Meanwhile, divide the lettuce leaves among 4 dinner plates. Top with the sliced cucumber. When the fritters are done, place 2 fritters on each leaf. Top with a dollop of mayonnaise, sprinkle with sliced green onions, and serve!

PER 2 WRAPS

Calories: 612 | Calories From Fat: 499 | Total Fat: 55.5g | Saturated Fat: 7.6g | Cholesterol: 192mg Sodium: 731mg | Carbs: 5.5g | Dietary Fiber: 1.9g | Net Carbs: 3.6g | Sugars: 1.8g | Protein: 22.5g

Greek-Style Sea Bass

Prep time: 5 minutes | Cook time:20 minutes | Serves 4

- 4 (5-oz) sea bass fillets
- 1 small onion, diced
- ½ cup vegetable broth
- 1 cup canned diced tomatoes
- ½ cup chopped black olives
- 2 tbsp capers, drained
- 2 cups packed spinach
- 2 tbsp extra-virgin olive oil
- Sea salt and pepper to taste
- 1 tsp Greek oregano

1. Preheat your oven to 375°F.
2. Coat the fish with olive oil in a baking dish Season with Greek oregano, salt, and pepper.
3. Top the fish with the onion, broth, tomatoes, olives, capers, spinach, salt, and pepper.
4. Cover the baking dish with aluminum foil and place it in the oven.
5. Bake for 15 minutes, or until the fish is cooked through.
6. Serve.

PER SERVING

Cal 275| Fat 12g| Carbs 5g| Protein 34g

Saucy Tropical Halibut

Prep time: 5 minutes | Cook time:30 minutes | Serves 4

- ½ mango, diced
- 1 avocado, diced
- ½ cup chopped strawberries
- 1 tsp chopped fresh mint
- 1 lemon, juiced and zested
- 1 tbsp olive oil
- 4 boneless, skinless halibut fillets
- Sea salt and pepper to taste

1. Mix avocado, mango, strawberries, mint, lemon juice, and lemon zest in a bowl| stir well.
2. Set the sauce aside.
3. Warm the olive oil in a pan over medium heat.
4. Lightly season the halibut with salt and pepper.
5. Add the fish and fry for 3-4 minutes per side, turning once or until it is just cooked through.
6. Top with avocado salsa and serve.

PER SERVING

Cal 355| Fat 15g| Carbs 12g| Protein 42g

Fish Taco Bowl

Prep time: 8 minutes | Cook time: 8 minutes | Serves 1

- 1 tablespoon avocado oil or other light-tasting oil, for the pan
- 1 (6-ounce) firm white fish fillet
- ½ teaspoon Cajun Seasoning
- ½ cup shredded green cabbage
- ¼ cup shredded red cabbage
- ½ medium cucumber, sliced
- ½ Hass avocado, sliced
- For garnish:
- ½ tablespoon chopped fresh cilantro
- 1½ teaspoons finely chopped red onions
- 2 lime wedges

1. Heat the oil in a medium-sized nonstick skillet for 2 minutes. Season the fish fillet on both sides with the Cajun seasoning.
2. Place the fish fillet in the hot oil and cook for 3 minutes per side, or until golden brown and cooked through. Remove the fish to a serving bowl.
3. Arrange the cabbage, cucumbers, and avocado slices around the fillet. Garnish with the cilantro, onions, and lime wedges before serving.

PER SERVING

Calories: 367 | Fat: 21g | Protein: 37g | Carbs: 12g | Fiber: 7g | Net Carbs: 5g

Seared Trout with Greek Yogurt Sauce

Prep time: 5 minutes | Cook time:25 minutes | Serves 4

- 1 garlic clove, minced
- 2 dill pickles, cubed
- ¼ cup Greek yogurt
- 3 tbsp olive oil
- 4 trout fillets, patted dry
- 1 tbsp olive oil
- Sea salt and pepper to taste

1. Whisk yogurt, pickles, garlic, 1 tbsp of olive oil, and salt in a small bowl.
2. Set the sauce aside.
3. Season the trout fillets lightly with salt and pepper.
4. Heat the remaining olive oil in a skillet over medium heat.
5. Add the trout fillets to the hot skillet and panfry for about 10 minutes, flipping the fish halfway through or until the fish is cooked to your liking.
6. Spread the salsa on top of the fish and serve.

PER SERVING

Cal 325| Fat 15g| Carbs 5g| Protein 38g

Shrimp Fajitas

Prep time: 15 minutes | Cook time: 6 minutes | Serves 4

- 1 tablespoon avocado oil or other light-tasting oil, for the pan
- 1 cup sliced red bell peppers
- 1 cup sliced yellow bell peppers
- ½ cup sliced red onions
- ¼ cup seeded and julienned jalapeño peppers
- 1 tablespoon ground cumin
- 1 teaspoon chipotle powder
- 1 teaspoon ground coriander
- 1 teaspoon kosher salt
- 1 teaspoon minced garlic
- ½ teaspoon ground paprika
- ¼ teaspoon ground black pepper
- 1 pound extra-large shrimp, peeled and deveined
- 2 tablespoons chopped fresh cilantro, plus more for garnish
- For The Avocado Crema:
- ¼ cup full-fat sour cream
- 2 tablespoons salsa verde
- ½ cup chopped avocado
- 2 batches Cream Cheese Wraps, for serving

1. Heat the oil in a large sauté pan over high heat. Add the bell peppers, onions, and jalapeño slices and sauté for 2 minutes, or until starting to brown.
2. Lower the heat to medium and add the cumin, chipotle powder, coriander, salt, garlic, paprika, and pepper and cook for 1 minute, or until fragrant and sizzling.
3. Add the shrimp and cook for 3 minutes, or until they have just turned white and pink; don't overcook the shrimp or they will be tough and dry. Remove from the heat and stir in the cilantro.
4. Make the avocado crema: Place the sour cream, salsa verde, and avocado in a small blender and blend for 30 seconds, or until smooth.
5. Assemble the fajitas: Divide the shrimp mixture among the 8 wraps and top with a generous drizzle of avocado crema. Garnish with some chopped cilantro and serve immediately.
6. The shrimp mixture, avocado crema, and wraps can be stored separately in the refrigerator for up to 5 days. Reheat the wraps for 15 seconds in the microwave before using. Reheat the shrimp mixture for 1 minute before assembling and serving.

PER SERVING

Calories: 376 | Fat: 17g | Protein: 29g | Carbs: 10g | Fiber: 3g | Net Carbs: 7g

Tarragon Scallops

Prep time: 5 minutes | Cook time:5minutes | Serves 1

- 2 garlic cloves, minced
- 1 red chili, minced
- 8 king scallops
- 1 tbsp olive oil
- Juice of ½ lime
- 2 tbsp chopped tarragon

1. Warm the olive oil in a skillet over medium heat and fry scallops for about 1 minute per side until lightly golden.
2. Add the chopped chili and garlic cloves to the pan and squeeze the lime juice over the scallops.
3. Saute for 2-3 minutes.
4. Sprinkle the tarragon over the top and serve.

PER SERVING

Cal 235| Fat 15g| Carbs 13g| Protein 15g

Creamy Lobster Risotto

Prep time: 15 minutes | Cook time: 18 minutes | Serves 2

- 3 cups salted filtered water
- 3 (4-ounce) lobster tails
- 2 tablespoons butter
- 3 cups riced cauliflower (see)
- ½ teaspoon kosher salt
- ¼ teaspoon ground black pepper
- ⅓ cup dry sherry
- 2 ounces mascarpone cheese (¼ cup)
- ¼ cup grated Parmesan cheese
- 2 tablespoons chopped scallions, plus more for garnish

1. Bring the water to a boil in a medium-sized saucepan. Add the lobster tails and boil for 5 minutes. Remove the lobster tails from the water and let cool. Reserve ¼ cup of the cooking water.
2. Remove the lobster meat from the tails and slice in half lengthwise (reserve two of the lobster tail shells for garnish, if desired). Keep two of the lobster tail halves intact for garnish and chop the other four halves into bite-sized pieces.
3. Melt the butter in a large sauté pan over medium heat. Add the riced cauliflower, salt, and pepper. Cook for 3 minutes, or until the cauliflower is starting to soften. Add the sherry and reserved lobster broth and cook for 3 minutes, or until the liquid is mostly absorbed. Stir in the mascarpone, Parmesan, scallions, and chopped lobster and cook for 2 more minutes.
4. Remove from the heat and divide between 2 serving bowls. Top each bowl with a lobster tail half, set inside the reserved shell, if desired. Garnish with additional chopped scallions and serve immediately.

PER SERVING

Calories: 449 | Fat: 30g | Protein: 11g | Carbs: 8g | Fiber: 3g | Net Carbs: 5g

One-Skillet Shrimp with Sriracha Pak Choy

Prep time: 5 minutes | Cook time:20 minutes | Serves 4

- ¼ cup olive oil
- 1½ lb peeled shrimp
- Sea salt and pepper to taste
- 4 cups pak choi, chopped
- 2 garlic cloves, minced
- ½ cup orange juice
- 1 tbsp sriracha sauce

1. Warm 2 tbsp of olive oil in a skillet over medium heat and place the shrimp and salt.
2. Cook for 4 minutes until the shrimp is pink.
3. Set aside covered with aluminum foil.
4. Warm 2 tbsp of olive oil in the skillet, add the pak choy, and cook for 3 minutes.
5. Stir in garlic and cook for another 30 seconds.
6. Mix the orange juice, Sriracha sauce, salt, and pepper in a bowl, pour it over the spinach, and cook for 3 more minutes.
7. Top shrimp and serve.

PER SERVING

Cal 320| Fat 17g| Carbs 8g| Protein 1g

Spicy Shrimp Stuffed Avocados

Prep time: 5 minutes, plus 10 minutes to chill | Cook time: 15 minutes | Serves 4

- 1 pound large shrimp, peeled, deveined, and cooked (tails removed)
- ⅓ cup sugar-free mayonnaise
- 2 tablespoons Sriracha sauce
- 1 teaspoon chopped fresh cilantro, plus more for garnish if desired
- 1 teaspoon lime juice
- 2 large ripe Hass avocados

1. Chop the shrimp into bite-sized pieces and place in a medium-sized bowl.
2. Add the mayonnaise, Sriracha, cilantro, and lime juice. Mix until well combined. Place in the refrigerator to chill for 10 minutes.
3. Just before serving, cut the avocados in half and remove the pits. Spoon ½ cup of the spicy shrimp mixture into each avocado half. Serve immediately, garnished with extra cilantro, if desired. If not consuming it right away, store the spicy shrimp mixture in the refrigerator for up to 5 days.

PER SERVING

Calories: 334 | Fat: 29g | Protein: 15g | Carbs: 8g | Fiber: 5g | Net Carbs: 3g

Fish Stew

Prep time: 5 minutes | Cook time:25 minutes | Serves 4

- 2 lb white fish fillets, cut into 2-inch pieces
- 1 white onion, sliced thin
- 1 fennel bulb, sliced thin
- 2 garlic cloves, minced
- 1 (28-oz) can diced tomatoes
- 2 tbsp extra-virgin olive oil
- ¼ tsp turmeric
- 1 tsp ground cumin
- 1 tsp ground oregano
- Sea salt and pepper to taste
- 2 tbsp chopped parsley
- ½ lemon, juiced

1. Warm the olive oil in a large pot over medium heat.
2. Add the onion, fennel, and garlic.
3. Sauté for 5 minutes.
4. Stir in the crushed tomatoes, turmeric, cumin, oregano, salt, and pepper.
5. Bring the mixture to a simmer.
6. Lay the fish fillets in a single layer over the vegetables, cover the pan, and simmer for 10 minutes.
7. Garnish with parsley and lemon juice.
8. Serve and enjoy!

PER SERVING

Cal 530| Fat 20g| Carbs 24g| Protein 61g

Lime Salmon Burgers

Prep time: 5 minutes | Cook time:25 minutes | Serves 4

- 2 tbsp olive oil
- 1 lime, cut into wedges
- 1 tsp garlic powder
- 1 scallion, chopped
- 1 lb cooked salmon fillet, flaked
- 2 eggs
- ¾ cup almond flour
- 1 lime, juiced and zested
- 1 tbsp chopped dill
- A pinch of sea salt

1. Combine the salmon, eggs, almond flour, garlic powder, scallion, lime juice, lime zest, dill, and salt in a large bowl and mix until the mixture holds together when pressed.
2. Divide the salmon mixture into 4 equal portions, and press them into patties about ½ inch thick.
3. Refrigerate them for about 30 minutes to firm up.
4. Warm the olive oil in a skillet over medium heat.
5. Add the salmon patties and brown for about 5 minutes per side, turning once.
6. Serve the patties with lime wedges.

PER SERVING

Cal 245| Fat 17g| Carbs 5g| Protein 19g

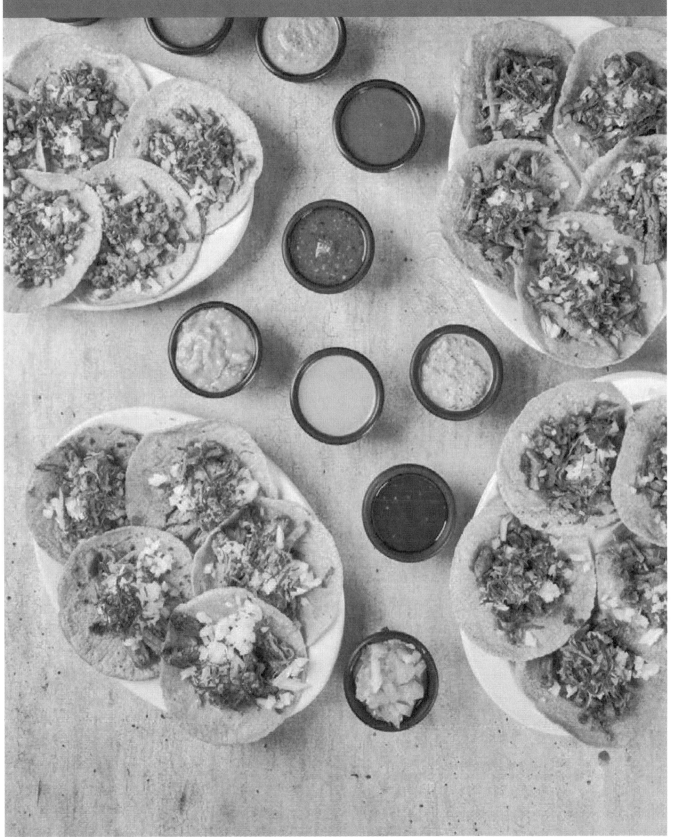

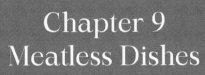

Chapter 9
Meatless Dishes

Celery & Turmeric Lentils

Prep time: 5 minutes | Cook time:15 minutes | Serves 4

- 2 tbsp olive oil
- 1 celery stalk, chopped
- 1 onion, chopped
- 1 tbsp ground turmeric
- 1 tsp garlic powder
- 1 (14-oz) can lentils, drained
- 1 (14-oz) can diced tomatoes
- Sea salt and pepper to taste

1. Warm the olive oil in a pot over medium heat and place the onion, celery, and turmeric.
2. Cook for 5 minutes until tender.
3. Stir in garlic powder, lentils, tomatoes, salt, and pepper and cook for 5 more minutes.
4. Serve immediately.

PER SERVING

Cal 250| Fat 9g| Carbs 35g| Protein 16g

Spaghetti with Tomato-Basil Sauce

Prep time: 5 minutes | Cook time:20 minutes | Serves 4

- 2 tbsp grated Parmesan
- 1 tbsp olive oil
- 1 onion, minced
- 2 garlic cloves, minced
- 2 (28-oz) cans diced tomatoes
- Sea salt and pepper to taste
- ¼ cup basil leaves, chopped
- 8 oz whole-wheat spaghetti

1. Warm the olive oil in a pot over medium heat, place the onion, and cook for 5 minutes until tender.
2. Stir in garlic and sauté for another 30 seconds.
3. Mix in tomatoes, salt, and pepper, bring to a simmer, and then low the heat and simmer for 5 minutes.
4. Turn the heat off and put the basil leaves.
5. Toss to combine.
6. Top with Parmesan and serve.

PER SERVING

Cal 340| Fat 9g| Carbs 57g| Protein 18g

Grandma's Black Bean Chili

Prep time: 5 minutes | Cook time:25 minutes | Serves 4

- 2 tbsp olive oil
- 1 tsp smoked paprika
- 1 onion, chopped
- 2 (28-oz) cans diced tomatoes
- 2 (14-oz) cans black beans
- 1 chili pepper, chopped
- 1 tsp garlic powder
- ½ tsp sea salt

1. Warm the olive oil in a pot over medium heat, place the onion, and cook for 5 minutes until tender.
2. Mix in tomatoes, black beans, chili pepper, garlic powder, smoked paprika, and salt and bring to a simmer.
3. Then low the heat and cook for 15 more minutes.
4. Serve warm.

PER SERVING

Cal 480| Fat 11g| Carbs 81g| Protein 20g

Buddha Bowl

Prep time: 10 minutes | Cook time: 20 minutes | Serves 4

- Nonstick coconut oil cooking spray
- 2 cups cubed butternut squash
- ⅓ cup coconut oil
- Sea salt
- Freshly ground black pepper
- 1 zucchini, spiralized or cut into noodles
- 1 cup chopped broccoli
- ½ cup edamame
- ⅓ cup sliced radishes
- ⅓ cup black olives
- 1 avocado, peeled, pitted, and sliced
- 1 tablespoon Tahini Goddess dressing
- Sesame seeds, for serving

1. Preheat the oven to 350°F. Grease a baking sheet with cooking spray and set aside.
2. In a large mixing bowl, toss the butternut squash in the coconut oil. Season with salt and pepper.
3. Arrange the squash on the prepared baking sheet and bake for 20 minutes until the squash is tender.
4. Remove the squash from the oven and place in the bottom of the serving bowl.
5. Top with the zucchini spirals, broccoli, edamame, radishes, olives, and avocado.
6. Garnish with the dressing and sprinkle with sesame seeds.

PER SERVING

Calories: 334 | Total Fat: 28g | Carbohydrates: 21g | Fiber: 8g | Net Carbs: 13g | Protein: 6g

Hurry Curry

Prep time: 10 minutes | Cook time: 35 minutes | Serves 6

- 1 tablespoon coconut oil
- 1 yellow onion, diced
- 2 tablespoons grated fresh ginger
- 2 garlic cloves, minced
- 3 tablespoons curry powder
- 1 tablespoon ground cumin
- 1 tablespoon tomato paste
- 2 cups chopped butternut squash
- 1 cup chopped broccoli
- 1 cup chopped red bell pepper
- 1 cup chopped eggplant
- 1 (4-ounce) can coconut cream
- ⅓ cup vegetable broth
- 4 cups fresh spinach
- 1 tablespoon chopped cilantro or Thai basil, for garnish

1. Heat the coconut oil in a large stockpot over medium-high heat.
2. Add the onion, ginger, and garlic to the pot. Cook until the onions become translucent and fragrant, about 3 minutes.
3. Stir in the curry powder, cumin, and tomato paste.
4. Add the squash, broccoli, bell pepper, and eggplant and stir a few times to coat the vegetables with the spices.
5. Stir in the coconut cream and vegetable broth.
6. Reduce the heat to low and simmer for 25 to 30 minutes to allow the curry to become thick and rich.
7. Remove the pot from the heat, add the spinach and cover the pot for a few minutes to let the spinach wilt.
8. Serve in bowls garnished with the cilantro or Thai basil.

PER SERVING

Calories: 133 | Total Fat: 8g | Carbohydrates: 17g | Fiber: 5g | Net Carbs: 12g | Protein: 3g

Keto Margherit-0 Pizza

Prep time: 10 minutes | Cook time: 25 minutes | Serves 4

- 1 cup lukewarm water
- ½ cup plus 2 tablespoons coconut flour
- 2 tablespoons ground psyllium husk
- ¼ teaspoon sea salt
- 1 tablespoon cold-pressed olive oil
- ¼ cup tomato sauce
- ¼ cup vegan mozzarella
- ¼ cup sliced mushrooms
- ¼ cup sliced olives
- ¼ cup fresh basil leaves, for garnish
- 1 teaspoon red pepper flakes, for garnish

1. Preheat the oven to 420°F. Prepare two pieces of parchment paper on a work surface. If you don't have parchment paper, use wax paper.
2. In a large mixing bowl, combine the water, coconut flour, psyllium husk, salt, and olive oil, and knead together to form the dough. If it's breaking apart, add more water a tablespoon at a time until the dough sticks together.
3. Set aside and allow the dough to rest for 10 minutes.
4. Turn the dough out onto one piece of parchment paper. Cover with the second piece and roll the dough out into a crust. A thinner crust will create a crisper texture.
5. Peel off the top layer of parchment paper. Leave the bottom piece of parchment paper intact to help slide the crust onto a baking sheet. Bake the crust for 15 minutes.
6. Remove the crust from the oven and top it with the tomato sauce, vegan mozzarella, mushrooms, and olives.
7. Return the pizza to the oven for a further 5 to 7 minutes until the cheese starts to toast and bubble.
8. Allow the pizza to cool for 10 minutes before cutting Cut with a rolling pizza slicer and serve garnished with the basil and red pepper flakes.

PER SERVING

Calories: 159 | Total Fat: 8g | Carbohydrates: 19g | Fiber: 11g | Net Carbs: 8g | Protein: 3g

Good Shepherd'S Pie

Prep time: 15 minutes | Cook time: 50 minutes | Serves 4

- For The Mashed Topping:
- 1 head cauliflower, coarsely chopped
- Sea salt
- ¼ cup cold-pressed olive oil
- ⅓ cup tahini
- White pepper
- For The Filling:
- Nonstick cooking spray
- 3 tablespoons cold-pressed olive oil, plus more for drizzling
- 1 yellow onion, chopped
- 1 shallot, chopped
- 2 garlic cloves, chopped
- 2 tablespoons white pepper
- 2 teaspoons onion powder
- 1 teaspoon fennel seeds
- 1 teaspoon ground coriander
- 1 teaspoon ground cumin
- ½ cup dry Marsala wine
- 5 cups chopped mushrooms
- 1 cup peas
- ½ cup chopped carrots
- ½ cup chopped celery
- ½ cup chopped walnuts
- ½ cup nutritional yeast
- 3 cups mushroom broth
- 1 thyme sprig
- 1 rosemary sprig, plus more, chopped, for garnish
- 3 cups fresh spinach

TO MAKE THE MASHED TOPPING:

1. Preheat the oven to 375°F.
2. Bring a large pot of water to a boil over high heat. Add the cauliflower and cook for about 12 minutes or until tender.
3. When cooked, the cauliflower should be so tender that it falls apart easily with a fork. Strain it and return it to the pot.
4. Add the olive oil and tahini and season with salt and white pepper. Mash with a potato masher, or for a creamier finish, whip with an immersion blender. Set aside.

TO MAKE THE FILLING:

1. While the cauliflower is cooking, Grease a 9-by-13-inch casserole dish with cooking spray.
2. In a large skillet over medium heat, warm the oil.
3. Add the onion, shallot, and garlic, white pepper, onion powder, fennel, coriander, and cumin to the skillet. Cook until the onions become tender and the spices are fragrant, about 5 minutes.
4. Pour in the Marsala wine to deglaze the pan. Allow the wine to cook off partially, 3 to 4 minutes.
5. Add the mushrooms, peas, carrots, celery, walnuts, and nutritional yeast, and stir to coat the vegetables in the spices.
6. Add the mushroom broth, plus the thyme and rosemary sprigs and simmer for about 20

minutes, until the sauce thickens and reduces.

TO ASSEMBLE THE PIE:

1. Arrange the vegetable mixture in an even layer in the prepared casserole dish.
2. Lay the spinach over the vegetables.
3. Top with the cauliflower mash, spreading it evenly to completely cover the spinach layer.
4. Top with a drizzle of olive oil and a sprinkle of rosemary and place in the oven to bake for 25 minutes.
5. Remove from the oven after the top starts to toast. Allow to cool for 10 minutes before serving To serve, cut into even-sized squares and plate.

PER SERVING

Calories: 615 | Total Fat: 46g | Carbohydrates: 37g | Fiber: 14g | Net Carbs: 23g | Protein: 24g

Shirataki Noodles Carbonara

Prep time: 5 minutes | Cook time: 15 minutes | Serves 4

- 1 (8-ounce) package shirataki noodles
- 4 tablespoons cold-pressed olive oil
- ½ yellow onion, chopped
- 1 cup sliced mushrooms
- 4 garlic cloves, chopped
- 1½ cups Vegan "Sour Cream"
- ¼ cup nutritional yeast, plus more for serving
- ½ cup dry white wine
- ½ cup peas
- Freshly ground black pepper
- ⅓ cup Coconut "Bacon"
- ¼ cup fresh basil, for garnish

1. Cook the noodles according to the package instructions, and set aside.
2. In a large skillet over medium-high heat, heat the olive oil.
3. Add the onion, mushrooms, and garlic, stirring regularly to prevent burning
4. Add the "sour cream," nutritional yeast, and white wine, and cook, stirring often, until the wine cooks off and the sauce reduces, about 5 minutes.
5. Add the peas and sauté for 3 minutes until they start to become tender.
6. Taste the sauce and season with pepper to taste.
7. Add the cooked noodles to the skillet, stirring often and allowing them to soak up the sauce for about 3 minutes.
8. Remove from the heat and plate the noodles. Top with the coconut "bacon," basil, more pepper, and a dusting of nutritional yeast.

PER SERVING

Calories: 530 | Total Fat: 46g | Carbohydrates: 23g | Fiber: 8g | Net Carbs: 15g | Protein: 19g

Warming Spiced Chili

Prep time: 5 minutes | Cook time: 1 hour | Serves 4

- 4 tablespoons cold-pressed olive oil
- 1 yellow onion, chopped
- 4 tablespoons chili powder
- 1 teaspoon ground cumin
- 1 teaspoon dried oregano
- 1 teaspoon ground allspice
- ½ teaspoon ground cinnamon
- 1 teaspoon ground coriander
- 2 thyme sprigs
- 1 can black soybeans, rinsed and drained
- ½ cup chopped walnuts
- ¼ cup hemp seeds
- 2 cups vegetable broth
- 1 (8-ounce) can chunky stewed tomatoes
- 3 tablespoons tomato paste
- 2 cups chopped fresh kale
- ½ cup chopped scallions, for garnish
- Cayenne pepper (optional)

1. In a large stockpot over medium heat, heat the olive oil.
2. Add the onion, chili powder, cumin, oregano, allspice, cinnamon, coriander, and thyme. Cook, stirring regularly, until the onion is tender, about 5 minutes.
3. Add the soybeans, walnuts, hemp seeds, vegetable broth, stewed tomatoes, and tomato paste. Reduce the heat to low and simmer for 45 minutes to allow the chili to thicken and the flavors to meld.
4. Stir in the kale and simmer for 4 more minutes.
5. Remove the chili from the heat and divide equally among small serving bowls.
6. Garnish with the scallions and some cayenne pepper if you want to add a little heat.

PER SERVING

Calories: 366 | Total Fat: 31g | Carbohydrates: 20g | Fiber: 9g | Net Carbs: 11g | Protein: 10g

Chipotle Kidney Bean Chili

Prep time: 5 minutes | Cook time:20 minutes | Serves 4

- 2 tbsp olive oil
- 1 onion, chopped
- 2 garlic cloves, minced
- 1 (16-oz) can tomato sauce
- 1 tbsp chili powder
- 1 chipotle chili, minced
- ½ tsp dried marjoram
- 1 (15.5-oz) can kidney beans
- Sea salt and pepper to taste
- ½ tsp cayenne pepper

1. Heat the oil in a pot over medium heat.
2. Place in onion and garlic and sauté for 3 minutes.
3. Put in tomato sauce, chipotle chili, chili powder, cumin, cayenne pepper, marjoram, salt, and pepper and cook for 5 minutes.
4. Stir in kidney beans and 2 cups of water.
5. Bring to a boil, then lower the heat and simmer for 15 minutes, stirring often.

PER SERVING

Cal 260| Fat 11g| Carbs 37g| Protein 6g

White Pizza with Mixed Mushrooms

Prep time: 5 minutes | Cook time:30 minutes | Serves 4

- 2 oz mixed mushrooms, sliced
- 2 eggs, beaten
- ½ cup paleo mayonnaise
- ¾ cup almond flour
- 1 tbsp psyllium husk powder
- 1 tsp baking powder
- 1 tbsp basil pesto
- 2 tbsp olive oil
- Sea salt and pepper to taste
- ½ cup coconut cream
- ¾ cup grated Parmesan
- Preheat your oven to 350°F.

1. In a bowl, add the eggs, mayonnaise, almond flour, psyllium husk powder, baking powder, and salt and whisk well.
2. Allow sitting for 5 minutes.
3. Pour the batter into a baking sheet and spread out with a spatula.
4. Bake for 10 minutes.
5. In a bowl, mix mushrooms with pesto, olive oil, salt, and black pepper.
6. Remove the crust from the oven and spread the coconut cream on top.
7. Add the mushroom mixture and Parmesan cheese.
8. Bake the pizza further until the cheese has melted, 5-10 minutes.
9. Serve sliced.

PER SERVING

Cal 430| Fat 30g| Carbs 27g| Protein 15g

Ginger-Lime Veggie Stir Fry

Prep time: 10 minutes | Cook time: 15 minutes | Serves 4

- 3 tablespoons coconut oil
- ⅓ cup minced scallions, plus more for serving
- 3 garlic cloves, chopped
- 1-inch knob ginger root, peeled and grated
- ½ cup diced butternut squash
- ½ cup diced celery
- ½ cup peas
- ½ cup ribbon-sliced red cabbage
- ¼ cup tamari, plus more for serving
- 1 tablespoon sesame oil
- Juice of 1 lime, divided
- 4 cups cauliflower rice
- 1 teaspoon chili oil

1. In a large skillet on medium heat, heat the coconut oil.
2. When the oil is warm, add the scallions and sauté until translucent, about 3 minutes.
3. Add the garlic and ginger, and cook, stirring often, until fragrant.
4. Stir in the squash, celery, peas, cabbage, tamari, sesame oil, and half the lime juice.
5. Stir-fry until the vegetables become slightly tender, about 10 minutes.
6. Add the cauliflower rice and remaining lime juice and cook for a further 5 minutes.
7. Remove from the heat and garnish with another splash of tamari, some chopped scallions, and the chili oil.

PER SERVING

Calories: 198 | Total Fat: 15g | Carbohydrates: 13g | Fiber: 4g | Net Carbs: 9g | Protein: 6g

Bean & Spinach Casserole

Prep time: 5 minutes | Cook time:30 minutes | Serves 6

- ½ cup whole-wheat breadcrumbs
- 1 (15.5-oz) can Great Northern beans
- 1 (15.5-oz) can Navy beans
- 3 tbsp olive oil
- 1 onion, chopped
- 2 carrots, chopped
- 1 celery stalk, chopped
- 2 garlic cloves, minced
- 1 cup baby spinach
- 3 tomatoes, chopped
- 1 cup vegetable broth
- 1 tbsp parsley, chopped
- 1 tsp dried thyme
- Sea salt and pepper to taste

1. Preheat your oven to 380°F.
2. Heat the oil in a skillet over medium heat.
3. Place in onion, carrots, celery, and garlic.
4. Sauté for 5 minutes.
5. Remove into a greased casserole.
6. Add in beans, spinach, tomatoes, broth, parsley, thyme, salt, and pepper and stir to combine.
7. Cover with foil and bake in the oven for 15 minutes.
8. Take out the casserole from the oven, remove the foil, and spread the breadcrumbs all over.
9. Bake for another 10 minutes until the top is crispy and golden.
10. Serve warm.

PER SERVING

Cal 320| Fat 8g| Carbs 49g| Protein 16g

Vegetable Tempura

Prep time: 17 minutes | Cook time: 5 minutes | Serves 4

- ½ cup coconut flour + extra for dredging
- Salt and black pepper to taste
- 3 egg yolks
- 2 red bell peppers, cut into strips
- 1 squash, peeled and cut into strips
- 1 broccoli, cut into florets
- 1 cup Chilled water
- Olive oil for frying
- Lemon wedges to serve
- Sugar-free soy sauce to serve

1. In a deep frying pan or wok, heat the olive oil over medium heat. Beat the eggs lightly with ½ cup of coconut flour and water. The mixture should be lumpy. Dredge the vegetables lightly in some flour, shake off the excess flour, dip it in the batter, and then into the hot oil.
2. Fry in batches for 1 minute each, not more, and remove with a perforated spoon onto a wire rack. Sprinkle with salt and pepper and serve with the lemon wedges and soy sauce.

PER SERVING

Kcal: 218 | Fat: 17g | Net Carbs: 0.9g | Protein: 3g

Cabbage & Bean Stir-Fry

Prep time: 5 minutes | Cook time:15 minutes | Serves 2

- 2 tbsp peanuts, chopped
- 1 cup cooked white beans
- 1 tsp olive oil
- 2 carrots, julienned
- 1 cup sliced red cabbage
- 1 red bell pepper, sliced
- 2 scallions, chopped
- 3 tbsp mint, chopped
- 1 cup bean sprouts
- ¼ cup peanut sauce
- ¼ cup cilantro, chopped
- 2 lime wedges

1. Heat oil in a skillet and cook carrots, cabbage, and bell pepper for 10-15 minutes.
2. Stir in scallions, mint, and bean sprouts and cook for 1-2 minutes.
3. Remove to a bowl.
4. Mix in white beans and peanut sauce| toss to combine.
5. Garnish with cilantro and peanuts.
6. Serve with lime wedges on the side.

PER SERVING

Cal 405| Fat 14g| Carbs 57g| Protein 96g

Pasta Primavera with Cherry Tomatoes

Prep time: 5 minutes | Cook time:20 minutes | Serves 4

- 8 oz whole-wheat fidelini
- 2 tbsp olive oil
- ½ tsp paprika
- 1 small red onion, sliced
- 2 garlic cloves, minced
- 1 cup dry white wine
- Sea salt and pepper to taste
- 18 cherry tomatoes, halved
- 1 lemon, zested and juiced
- 1 cup basil leaves

1. Heat the olive oil in a pot.
2. Add the paprika, onion, garlic, and stir-fry for 2-3 minutes.
3. Mix in white wine, pasta, salt, and pepper.
4. Cover with water.
5. Cook until the water absorbs and the fidelini al dente, 5 minutes.
6. Mix in cherry tomatoes, lemon zest, lemon juice, and basil.
7. Serve.

PER SERVING

Cal 365| Fat 14g| Carbs 49g| Protein 11g

Garlic Fried Cauliflower Rice

Prep time: 10 minutes | Cook time: 20 minutes | Serves 4

- 1 (14-ounce) block sprouted tofu
- 4 tablespoons nutritional yeast
- 2 tablespoons tahini
- 1 teaspoon kala namak salt
- 1 teaspoon turmeric powder
- 1 tablespoon sesame oil
- 1 shallot, chopped
- 2 garlic cloves, chopped
- 1 tablespoon ground ginger
- 1 cup chopped carrots
- 1 cup peas
- 6 cups cauliflower rice
- ½ cup chopped scallions, plus more for garnish
- ¼ cup tamari, plus more for drizzling

1. Drain the tofu, pressing it with a paper towel to absorb as much water as possible.
2. In a medium mixing bowl, crumble the tofu and mix it with the nutritional yeast, tahini, turmeric, and kala namak to create an egg-like texture.
3. In a large skillet over medium heat, heat the sesame oil and add the shallot, garlic, and ginger, and cook, stirring regularly to prevent burning, until fragrant, about 3 minutes.
4. Add the carrots and peas and cook until the carrots become slightly tender, about 5 minutes.
5. Add the tofu "eggs" to the skillet and toss. Allow the tofu to toast up slightly on each side.
6. Add the cauliflower rice, scallions, and tamari and stir thoroughly to mix all the flavors.
7. Cook for 5 minutes to allow the flavors to meld and any excess liquid to cook off.
8. Remove from the heat, drizzle with a splash of tamari, and garnish with chopped scallions.

PER SERVING

Calories: 288 | Total Fat: 13g | Carbohydrates: 26g | Fiber: 9g | Net Carbs: 17g | Protein: 23g

Lemony Green Bean Risotto

Prep time: 5 minutes | Cook time:20 minutes | Serves 4

- 2 tsp almond butter
- 2 cloves minced garlic
- 1 cup brown rice
- 2 cups vegetable broth
- 2 cups green beans
- 2 tbsp parsley, chopped

1. Melt the almond butter in a skillet over medium heat.
2. Place in garlic and cook for 1 minute.
3. Stir in rice, broth, salt, and pepper.
4. Bring to a boil, then lower the heat and simmer for 10 minutes.
5. Put in the green beans and cook for another 10 minutes.
6. Fluff the rice with a fork and sprinkle with parsley.
7. Serve and enjoy!

PER SERVING

Cal 210| Fat 3g| Carbs 42g| Protein 1g

Cremini Mushroom Stroganoff

Prep time: 25 minutes | Cook time: 13 minutes | Serves 4

- 3 tbsp butter
- 1 white onion, chopped
- 4 cups cremini mushrooms, cubed
- 2 cups water
- ½ cup heavy cream
- ½ cup grated Parmesan cheese
- 1 ½ tbsp dried mixed herbs
- Salt and black pepper to taste

1. Melt the butter in a saucepan over medium heat and sauté the onion for 3 minutes until soft.
2. Stir in the mushrooms and cook until tender, about 5 minutes. Add the water, mix, and bring to boil for 10-15 minutes until the water reduces slightly.
3. Pour in the heavy cream and Parmesan cheese. Stir to melt the cheese. Also, mix in the dried herbs. Season with salt and black pepper, simmer for 5 minutes and turn the heat off.
4. Ladle stroganoff over a bed of spaghet
5. ti squash and serve.

PER SERVING

Kcal: 284 | Fat: 28g | Net Carbs: 1,5g | Protein: 8g

Hot Coconut Beans with Vegetables

Prep time: 5 minutes | Cook time:15 minutes | Serves 4

- 2 tbsp olive oil
- 1 onion, chopped
- 1 red bell pepper, chopped
- 2 garlic cloves, minced
- 1 tbsp hot powder
- 1 (13.5-oz) can coconut milk
- 2 (15.5-oz) cans white beans
- 1 (14.5-oz) can diced tomatoes
- 3 cups fresh baby spinach
- Sea salt and pepper to taste
- Chopped toasted walnuts

1. Heat the oil in a pot over medium heat.
2. Place in onion, garlic, hot powder, and bell pepper and sauté for 5 minutes, stirring occasionally.
3. Put in the coconut milk and whisk until well mixed.
4. Add in white beans, tomatoes, spinach, salt, and pepper and cook for 5 minutes until the spinach wilts.
5. Garnish with walnuts and serve.

PER SERVING

Cal 690| Fat 52g| Carbs 48g| Fiber 9g

Stuffed Cremini Mushrooms

Prep time: 35 minutes | Cook time: 25 to 29 minutes | Serves 4

- ½ head broccoli, cut into florets
- pound cremini mushrooms, stems removed
- tbsp coconut oil
- 1 onion, chopped
- 1 tsp garlic, minced
- 1 bell pepper, chopped
- 1 tsp cajun seasoning
- Salt and black pepper, to taste
- 1 cup cheddar cheese, shredded

1. Use a food processor to pulse broccoli florets until become like small rice-like granules.
2. Set oven to 360°F. Bake mushroom caps until tender for 8 to 12 minutes. In a heavybottomed skillet, melt the oil; stir in bell pepper, garlic, and onion and sauté until fragrant. Place in black pepper, salt, and cajun seasoning. Fold in broccoli rice.
3. Equally separate the filling mixture among mushroom caps. Cover with cheddar cheese and bake for 17 more minutes. Serve warm.

PER SERVING

Kcal: 206 | Fat: 13.4g | Net Carbs: 10g | Protein: 12.7g

Vegetable Burritos

Prep time: 10 minutes | Cook time: 4 minutes | Serves 4

- 2 large low carb tortillas
- 2 tsp olive oil
- 1 small onion, sliced
- 1 bell pepper, seeded and sliced
- 1 large ripe avocado, pitted and sliced
- 1 cup lemon cauli couscous
- Salt and black pepper to taste
- ⅓ cup sour cream
- 3 tbsp Mexican salsa

1. Heat the olive oil in a skillet and sauté the onion and bell pepper until they start to brown on the edges, about 4 minutes. Turn the heat off and set the skillet aside.
2. Lay the tortillas on a flat surface and top each with the bell pepper mixture, avocado, cauli couscous, season with salt and black pepper, sour cream, and Mexican salsa. Fold in the sides of each tortilla, and roll them in and over the filling to be completely enclosed. Wrap with foil, cut in halves, and serve warm.

PER SERVING

Kcal: 373 | Fat: 23.2g | Net Carbs: 5.4g | Protein: 17.9g

Walnut Tofu Sauté

Prep time: 15 minutes | Cook time: 6 minutes | Serves 4

- 1 tbsp olive oil
- 1 (8 oz) block firm tofu, cubed
- 1 tbsp tomato paste with garlic and onion
- 1 tbsp balsamic vinegar
- Salt and black pepper to taste
- ½ tsp mixed dried herbs
- 1 cup chopped raw walnuts

1. Heat the oil in a skillet over medium heat and cook the tofu for 3 minutes while stirring to brown.
2. Mix the tomato paste with the vinegar and add to the tofu. Stir, season with salt and black pepper, and cook for another 4 minutes.
3. Add the herbs and walnuts. Stir and cook on low heat for 3 minutes to be fragrant. Spoon to a side of squash mash and a sweet berry sauce to serve.

PER SERVING

Kcal: 320 | Fat: 24g | Net Carbs: 4g | Protein: 18g

Wild Mushroom and Asparagus Stew

Prep time: 25 minutes | Cook time: 18 minutes | Serves 4

- 2 tbsp olive oil
- cup onions, chopped
- garlic cloves, pressed
- ½ cup celery, chopped
- 2 carrots, chopped
- cup wild mushrooms, sliced
- tbsp dry white wine
- 2 rosemary sprigs, chopped
- 1 thyme sprig, chopped
- 4 cups vegetable stock
- ½ tsp chili pepper
- tsp smoked paprika
- tomatoes, chopped
- 1 tbsp flax seed meal

1. Set a pot over medium heat and warm oil. Add in onions and cook until tender, about 3 minutes. Place in carrots, celery, and garlic and cook until soft for 4 more minutes. Add in mushrooms and cook until the liquid evaporates; then set aside. Stir in wine to deglaze the pot's bottom.
2. Place in thyme and rosemary. Pour in tomatoes, vegetable stock, paprika, and chili pepper; add in reserved vegetables and allow to boil. On low heat, allow the mixture to simmer for 15 minutes. Stir in flax seed meal to thicken the stew. Plate into individual bowls and serve.

PER SERVING

Kcal: 114 | Fat: 7.3g | Net Carbs: 9.5g | Protein: 2.1g | Fiber: 5g

Traditional Cilantro Pilaf

Prep time: 5 minutes | Cook time: 25 minutes | Serves 6

- 3 tbsp extra-virgin olive oil
- 1 onion, minced
- 1 carrot, chopped
- 2 garlic cloves, minced
- 1 cup wild rice
- 1½ tsp ground fennel seeds
- ½ tsp ground cumin
- Sea salt and pepper to taste
- 3 tbsp minced cilantro

1. Heat the oil in a pot over medium heat.
2. Add onion, carrot, and garlic and sauté for 5 minutes.
3. Stir in rice, fennel seeds, cumin, and 2 cups of water.
4. Bring to a boil, then lower the heat and simmer for 20 minutes.
5. Remove and fluff with a fork.
6. Top with cilantro and black pepper.

PER SERVING

Cal 170 | Fat 7g | Carbs 24g | Protein 5g | Fiber: 4g

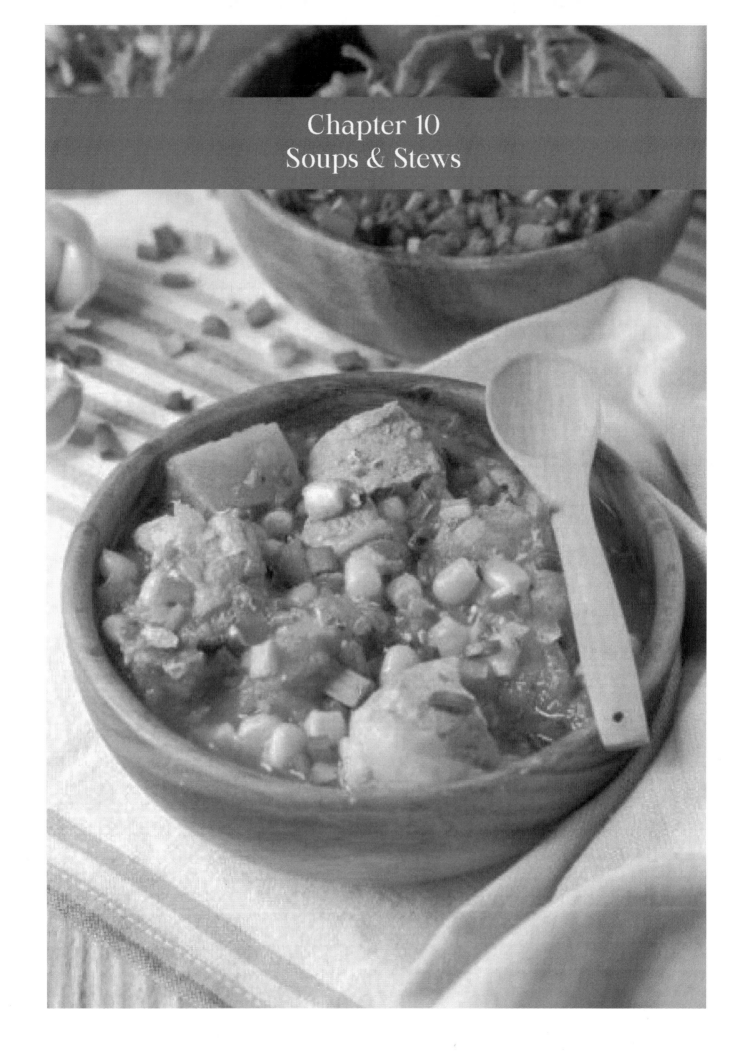

Chapter 10
Soups & Stews

Parsley Tomato Soup

Prep time: 5 minutes | Cook time:20 minutes | Serves 4

- 4 cups no-salt-added vegetable broth
- 2 tbsp parsley, chopped
- 2 tbsp extra-virgin olive oil
- 1 onion, finely chopped
- 2 garlic cloves, minced
- 2 (28-oz) cans diced tomatoes
- Sea salt and pepper to taste

1. Warm the olive oil in a pot over medium heat and place the onion.
2. Cook for 7 minutes until browned.
3. Add in garlic and cook for another 30 seconds.
4. Stir in tomatoes, vegetable broth, salt, and pepper and simmer for 5 minutes.
5. Puree the mixture with an immersion blender until smooth.
6. Serve warm topped with parsley.

PER SERVING

Cal 240| Fat 8g| Carbs 36g| Protein 11g| Fiber:5g

Celery & Sweet Potato Soup

Prep time: 5 minutes | Cook time:50 minutes | Serves 6

- 2 tbsp extra-virgin olive oil
- 1 onion, chopped
- 1 carrot, chopped
- 1 celery stalk, chopped
- 2 garlic cloves, minced
- 1 golden beet, diced
- 1 red bell pepper, chopped
- 1 sweet potato, diced
- 6 cups vegetable broth
- 1 tsp dried thyme
- Sea salt and pepper to taste
- 1 tbsp lemon juice

1. Heat the oil in a pot over medium heat.
2. Place the onion, carrot, celery, and garlic.
3. Cook for 5 minutes or until softened.
4. Stir in beet, bell pepper, and sweet potato, cook uncovered for 1 minute.
5. Pour in the broth and thyme.
6. Season with salt and pepper.
7. Cook for 45 minutes until the vegetables are tender.
8. Serve topped with lemon juice.

PER SERVING

Cal 100| Fat 5g| Carbs 14g| Protein 1g| Fiber:5g

Chicken & Vegetable Stew with Barley

Prep time: 5 minutes | Cook time:25 minutes | Serves 6

- 1 lb chicken breasts, cubed
- 3 tbsp extra-virgin olive oil
- 1 onion, chopped
- 2 garlic cloves, minced
- 2 turnips, chopped
- 1 cup pearl barley
- 1 (28-oz) can diced tomatoes
- 3 tsp dried mixed herbs
- Sea salt and pepper to taste

1. Warm the olive oil in a pot over medium heat.
2. Add the chicken, onion, and garlic and sauté for 6-8 minutes.
3. Stir in the turnips, barley, tomatoes, 3 cups of water, and herbs.
4. Cook for 20 minutes.
5. Adjust the seasoning.
6. Serve.

PER SERVING

Cal 350| Fat 15g| Carbs 36g| Protein 21g| Fiber:6g

Vegetable Soup with Vermicelli

Prep time: 5 minutes | Cook time:15 minutes | Serves 6

- 1 tbsp extra-virgin olive oil
- 1 onion, chopped
- 4 garlic cloves, minced
- 1 (14-oz) can diced tomatoes
- 6 cups vegetable broth
- 8 oz vermicelli
- 5 oz baby spinach

1. Warm the oil in a pot over medium heat.
2. Place in onion and garlic and cook for 3 minutes.
3. Stir in tomatoes, broth, salt, and pepper.
4. Bring to a boil, then lower the heat and simmer for 5 minutes.
5. Pour in vermicelli and spinach and cook for another 5 minutes.
6. Serve warm.

PER SERVING

Cal 180| Fat 3g| Carbs 39g| Protein 1g| Fiber:8g

Mushroom Curry Soup

Prep time: 5 minutes | Cook time:10minutes | Serves 4

- ½ cup sliced shiitake mushrooms
- 1 tbsp coconut oil
- 1 red onion, sliced
- 1 carrot, chopped
- 2 garlic cloves, minced
- 1 (13.5-oz) can coconut milk
- 4 cups vegetable stock
- 1 (8-oz) can tomato sauce
- 2 tbsp cilantro, chopped
- Juice from 1 lime
- Sea salt to taste
- 2 tbsp red curry paste

1. Melt coconut oil in a pot over medium heat.
2. Place in onion, garlic, carrot, and mushrooms and sauté for 5 minutes.
3. Pour in coconut milk, vegetable stock, tomato sauce, cilantro, lime juice, salt, and curry paste.
4. Cook until heated through.
5. Serve and enjoy!

PER SERVING

Cal 310| Fat 28g| Carbs 16g| Protein 2g| Fiber:5g

Green Bean & Rice Soup

Prep time: 5 minutes | Cook time:45 minutes | Serves 4

- 2 tbsp extra-virgin olive oil
- 1 medium onion, minced
- 2 garlic cloves minced
- ½ cup brown rice
- 1 cup green beans, chopped
- 2 tbsp chopped parsley

1. Heat oil in a pot over medium heat.
2. Place in onion and garlic and sauté for 3 minutes.
3. Add in rice, 4 cups water, salt, and pepper.
4. Bring to a boil, lower the heat, and simmer for 15 minutes.
5. Stir in beans and cook for 10 minutes.
6. Top with parsley.
7. Serve and enjoy!

PER SERVING

Cal 170| Fat 8g| Carbs 23g| Protein 1g| Fiber:4g

Beef & Enoki Mushroom Stew

Prep time: 5 minutes | Cook time:25 minutes | Serves 4

- 2 tbsp extra-virgin olive oil
- 1 tsp dried parsley
- 1 onion, chopped
- 1½ lb beef, cut into pieces
- 4 sweet potatoes, cubed
- 2 carrots, chopped
- 4 cups beef broth
- 1 cup diced enoki mushrooms

1. Heat the oil in the pressure cooker on "Sauté".
2. Add the meat and brown it on all sides.
3. Stir in the remaining ingredients.
4. Seal the lid and cook for 15 minutes on "Manual" on High pressure.
5. Do a quick pressure release, then perform a quick release.
6. Serve warm.

PER SERVING

Cal 527| Fat 15g| Carbs 50g| Protein 45g| Fiber:8g

Habanero Bean Soup with Brown Rice

Prep time: 5 minutes | Cook time:25 minutes | Serves 6

- ¼ cup sun-dried tomatoes, chopped
- 2 tbsp extra-virgin olive oil
- 3 garlic cloves, minced
- 1 tbsp chili powder
- 1 tsp dried oregano
- 1 (15.5-oz) can kidney beans
- 1 habanero pepper, chopped
- 6 cups vegetable broth
- Sea salt and pepper to taste
- ½ cup brown rice
- 1 tbsp chopped cilantro

1. Heat the oil in a pot over medium heat.
2. Place in garlic and sauté for 1 minute.
3. Add in chili powder, oregano, beans, habanero, tomatoes, broth, rice, salt, and pepper.
4. Cook for 20-30 minutes.
5. Garnish with cilantro to serve.

PER SERVING

Cal 285| Fat 6g| Carbs 46g| Protein 5g| Fiber:5

Chicken Vegetable Soup

Prep time: 5 minutes | Cook time: 45 minutes | Serves 8

- 2 tablespoons avocado oil
- 2 garlic cloves, minced
- ½ large onion, diced
- 1 bell pepper, diced
- 2 celery stalks, diced
- 1 (32-ounce) carton chicken bone broth
- 4 cups water
- 2 tablespoons apple cider vinegar
- 1 pound boneless, skinless chicken breasts
- 1 (15-ounce) can tomatoes with green chilies
- 2 cups green beans, fresh or frozen
- 1 teaspoon sea salt
- 2 bay leaves
- 1 small bunch fresh thyme
- 2 cups shredded kale

1. Heat the avocado oil in a large soup pot over medium heat. Sauté the garlic, onion, bell pepper, and celery for 5 minutes.
2. Add the bone broth, water, and vinegar. Stir well. Add the chicken, tomatoes, green beans, salt, bay leaves, and thyme.
3. Bring the soup to a boil, reduce the heat to low, and cover. Simmer for 25 minutes, or until the chicken has cooked through and the internal temperature reaches 165°F.
4. Carefully remove the chicken, shred it using two forks, and return it to the soup.
5. Remove the bay leaves and thyme, and stir in the kale. Add more sea salt to taste. When the kale has wilted a bit, the soup is ready to serve.

PER SERVING

Calories: 162 | Fat: 2.7g | Saturated Fat: 0.1g | Protein: 23.7g | Carbohydrate: 10.3g | Fiber: 2g | Sodium: 715mg

Lamb Stew

Prep time: 5 minutes | Cook time: 3 hours | Serves 6

- 4 cups lamb or chicken broth
- 4 cups water
- 1 (32-ounce) can crushed tomatoes
- 1 bouquet garni package (thyme, oregano, parsley, bay leaf), tied with twine
- 1 large red onion, diced
- 1 tablespoon grapeseed oil
- 3 lamb shanks
- 1 lemon, halved and seeded
- 1 cup black olives, pitted

1. In a large pot over medium-high heat, combine the broth, water, tomatoes, bouquet garni, and onion. Cover.
2. Heat the grapeseed oil in a large skillet over medium-high heat until shimmering. Add the lamb shanks and sear for 3 minutes on each side.
3. Add the seared lamb to the pot and bring almost to a boil. Reduce the heat to medium-low and simmer gently for 2 hours.
4. Squeeze the lemon juice directly into the pot. Add the lemon halves to the pot along with the olives. Cook uncovered for 15 minutes.
5. Remove from the heat and let the stew rest for 15 minutes.
6. Remove and discard the bouquet garni and lemon halves. Pull the meat from the bones. Discard the bones or save for making stock. Serve.

PER SERVING

Calories: 327 | Fat: 14.6g | Saturated Fat: 4.1g | Protein: 21.2g | Carbohydrate: 26.8g | Fiber: 8.4g | Sodium: 1613mg

Chicken Creamy Soup

Prep time: 15 minutes | Cook time: 5 minutes | Serves 4

- 2 cups cooked and shredded chicken
- 3 tbsp butter, melted
- 4 cups chicken broth
- 4 tbsp chopped cilantro ⅓ cup buffalo sauce
- ½ cup cream cheese
- Salt and black pepper, to taste

1. Blend the butter, buffalo sauce, and cream cheese, in a food processor, until smooth. Transfer to a pot, add chicken broth and heat until hot but do not bring to a boil.
2. Stir in chicken, salt, black pepper and cook until heated through. When ready, remove to soup bowls and serve garnished with cilantro.

PER SERVING

Kcal: 406 | Fat: 29.5g | Net Carbs: 5g | Protein: 26.5g | Fiber: 6g

Turkey Meatball Soup

Prep time: 5 minutes | Cook time: 1 hour, 10 minutes | Serves 8

MEATBALLS:

- 1 pound ground turkey
- 1 tablespoon coconut flour
- ½ cup finely chopped fresh parsley
- 2 large eggs
- ½ teaspoon sea salt
- ½ teaspoon garlic powder

SOUP:

- 4 tablespoons avocado oil
- 4 celery stalks, diced
- 1 sweet onion, diced
- 1 bell pepper, diced
- 2 garlic cloves, minced
- 1 (32-ounce) carton chicken stock
- 2 cups water
- 1 (28-ounce) can diced tomatoes
- 1 tablespoon Italian seasoning
- 1 teaspoon sea salt
- 2 cups shredded fresh kale or spinach
- ¼ cup finely chopped fresh parsley

1. Preheat the oven to 400°F. Line a baking sheet with parchment paper.
2. In a large bowl, combine all the meatball . Using clean hands, mix together well.
3. Scoop out tablespoonfuls of the meatball mixture, roll into balls, and place on the baking sheet, to make 40 small meatballs. Bake for 15 minutes, remove from the oven, and set aside.
4. Meanwhile, heat the avocado oil in a large soup pot over medium heat. Sauté the celery, onion, bell pepper, and garlic for 5 minutes, or until the vegetables are soft.
5. Pour in the chicken stock, water, tomatoes with their juice, Italian seasoning, and salt. Bring to a boil, reduce to a low simmer, and cover. Let the soup simmer for 30 to 45 minutes.
6. Remove the lid and add the cooked meatballs, kale, and parsley. Cook for 10 minutes, or until the meatballs are fully cooked through.

PER SERVING

Calories: 261 | Fat: 12.6g | Saturated Fat: 2.5g | Protein: 28.2g | Carbohydrate: 13.2g | Fiber: 4.4g | Sodium: 699mg

Sweet African Soup

Prep time: 5 minutes | Cook time: 40minutes | Serves 4

- 1 tbsp extra-virgin olive oil
- 1 onion, chopped
- 1 carrot, chopped
- 1 garlic clove, minced
- 3 Granny Smith apples, diced
- 2 tbsp curry powder
- 2 tsp tomato paste
- 3 cups vegetable broth
- Sea salt to taste
- 1 cup soy milk
- 4 tsp sugar-free apricot jam

1. Heat the olive oil in a pot over medium heat.
2. Place onion, carrot, and garlic and sauté for 5 minutes.
3. Stir in apples and cook for 5 minutes, until the apples soften.
4. Add in tomato paste, broth, and salt.
5. Cook for 10 minutes.
6. Blend the soup in a food processor until smooth.
7. Transfer to a bowl and mix with soy milk.
8. Close the lid and let chill in the fridge for 3 hours.
9. Serve topped with apricot jam.

PER SERVING

Cal 180| Fat 6g| Carbs 29g| Protein 4g

Spinach & Sweet Potato Lentil Soup

Prep time: 5 minutes | Cook time:50minutes | Serves 4

- 2 tbsp extra-virgin olive oil
- 1 onion, chopped
- 2 garlic cloves, minced
- 4 cups vegetable broth
- 2 sweet potatoes, cubed
- ½ tsp dried oregano
- ¼ tsp crushed red pepper
- Sea salt to taste
- 4 cups chopped spinach
- 1 cup green lentils, rinsed

1. Warm the oil in a pot over medium heat.
2. Place the onion and garlic and cook covered for 5 minutes.
3. Stir in broth, sweet potatoes, oregano, red pepper, lentils, and salt.
4. Bring to a boil, then lower the heat and simmer uncovered for 30 minutes.
5. Add in spinach and cook for another 5 minutes.
6. Serve immediately.

PER SERVING

Cal 95| Fat 5g| Carbs 11g| Protein 3g

Fall Medley Stew

Prep time: 5 minutes | Cook time:60 minutes | Serves 4

- 2 tbsp extra-virgin olive oil
- 8 oz seitan, cubed
- 1 leek, chopped
- 2 garlic cloves, minced
- 1 daikon, chopped
- 1 carrot, chopped
- 1 parsnip, chopped
- ½ lb butternut squash, cubed
- 1 head savoy cabbage, grated
- 1 (14.5-oz) can diced tomatoes
- 1 (15.5-oz) can white beans
- 2 cups vegetable broth
- ½ cup dry white wine
- ½ tsp dried thyme
- 4 oz crumbled angel hair pasta

1. Heat oil in a pot over medium heat.
2. Place in seitan and cook for 3 minutes.
3. Sprinkle with salt and pepper.
4. Add leek and garlic and cook for 3 minutes.
5. Stir in daikon, carrot, parsnip, and squash and cook for 10 minutes.
6. Add cabbage, tomatoes, white beans, broth, wine, thyme, salt, and pepper.
7. Bring to a boil and simmer for 15 minutes.
8. Put in pasta and cook for 5 minutes.
9. Serve.

PER SERVING

Cal 380| Fat 12g| Carbs 52g| Protein 28g

Broccoli Cheese Soup

Prep time: 20 minutes | Cook time: 1 minutes | Serves 4

- ¾ cup heavy cream 1 onion, diced
- 1 tsp minced garlic
- 4 cups chopped broccoli
- 4 cups veggie broth
- tbsp butter
- cups grated cheddar cheese
- Salt and black pepper, to taste
- ½ bunch fresh mint, chopped

1. Melt the butter in a large pot over medium heat. Sauté onion and garlic for 3 minutes or until tender, stirring occasionally. Season with salt and black pepper. Add the broth, broccoli and bring to a boil.
2. Reduce the heat and simmer for 10 minutes. Puree the soup with a hand blender until smooth. Add in 2 ¾ cups of the cheddar cheese and cook about 1 minute. Taste and adjust the seasoning. Stir in the heavy cream. Serve in bowls with the remaining cheddar cheese and sprinkled with fresh mint.

PER SERVING

Kcal: 561 | Fat: 52.3g | Net Carbs: 7g | Protein: 23.8g

Salsa Verde Chicken Soup

Prep time: 15 minutes | Cook time: 8 minutes | Serves 4

- ½ cup salsa verde
- 2 cups cooked and shredded chicken
- 2 cups chicken broth
- 1 cup shredded cheddar cheese
- 4 ounces cream cheese ½ tsp chili powder
- ½ tsp ground cumin
- ½ tsp fresh cilantro, chopped
- Salt and black pepper, to taste

1. Combine the cream cheese, salsa verde, and broth, in a food processor; pulse until smooth. Transfer the mixture to a pot and place over medium heat. Cook until hot, but do not bring to a boil. Add chicken, chili powder, and cumin and cook for about 3-5 minutes, or until it is heated through.
2. Stir in cheddar cheese and season with salt and pepper to taste. If it is very thick, add a few tablespoons of water and boil for 1-3 more minutes. Serve hot in bowls sprinkled with fresh cilantro.

PER SERVING

Kcal: 346 | Fat: 23g | Net Carbs: 3g | Protein: 25g

Pumpkin & Meat Peanut Stew

Prep time: 45 minutes | Cook time: 36 minutes | Serves 6

- 1 cup pumpkin puree
- 2 pounds chopped pork stew meat
- 1 tbsp peanut butter
- 4 tbsp chopped peanuts
- 1 garlic clove, minced ½ cup chopped onion
- ½ cup white wine 1 tbsp olive oil
- tsp lemon juice
- ¼ cup granulated sweetener
- ¼ tsp cardamom powder
- ¼ tsp allspice
- cups water
- 2 cups chicken stock

1. Heat the olive oil in a large pot and sauté onion for 3 minutes, until translucent. Add garlic and cook for 30 more seconds. Add the pork and cook until browned, about 5-6 minutes, stirring occasionally. Pour in the wine and cook for one minute.
2. Add in the remaining ingredients, except for the lemon juice and peanuts. Bring the mixture to a boil, and cook for 5 minutes. Reduce the heat to low, cover the pot, and let cook for about 30 minutes. Adjust seasonings and stir in the lemon juice before serving.
3. Ladle into bowls and serve topped with peanuts.

PER SERVING

Kcal: 451 | Fat: 33g | Net Carbs: 4g | Protein: 27.5g

Creamy Cauliflower Soup with Chorizo Sausage

Prep time: 40 minutes | Cook time: 34 minutes | Serves 4

- 1 cauliflower head, chopped
- 1 turnip, chopped
- 3 tbsp butter
- chorizo sausage, sliced
- cups chicken broth
- small onion, chopped
- cups water
- Salt and black pepper, to taste

1. Melt 2 tbsp of the butter in a large pot over medium heat. Stir in onion and cook until soft and golden, about 3-4 minutes.
2. Add cauliflower and turnip, and cook for another 5 minutes. Pour the broth and water over. Bring to a boil, simmer covered, and cook for about 20 minutes until the vegetables are tender. Remove from heat. Melt the remaining butter in a skillet. Add the chorizo sausage and cook for 5 minutes until crispy.
3. Puree the soup with a hand blender until smooth. Taste and adjust the seasonings. Serve the soup in deep bowls topped with the chorizo sausage.

PER SERVING

Kcal: 251 | Fat: 19.1g | Net Carbs: 5.7g | Protein: 10g

Coconut Artichoke Soup with Almonds

Prep time: 5 minutes | Cook time:25 minutes | Serves 4

- 1 tbsp extra-virgin olive oil
- 2 medium shallots, chopped
- 10 oz artichoke hearts
- 3 cups vegetable broth
- 1 tsp fresh lemon juice
- Sea salt to taste
- 2 tbsp olive oil
- ⅛ tsp cayenne pepper
- 1 cup plain coconut cream
- 1 tbsp snipped fresh chives
- 2 tbsp toasted almond slices

1. Heat the oil in a pot over medium heat.
2. Place in shallots and sauté until softened, about 3 minutes.
3. Add in artichokes, broth, lemon juice, and salt.
4. Bring to a boil, lower the heat, and simmer for 10 minutes.
5. Stir in cayenne pepper.
6. Transfer to a food processor and blend until purée.
7. Return to the pot.
8. Mix in coconut cream and simmer for 5 minutes.
9. Top with chives and almonds.

PER SERVING

Cal 450 | Fat 43g | Carbs 17g | Protein 5g

Thyme & Wild Mushroom Soup

Prep time: 25 minutes | Cook time: 20 minutes | Serves 4

- ¼ cup butter
- ½ cup crème fraiche
- 12 oz wild mushrooms, chopped
- 2 tsp thyme leaves
- 2 garlic cloves, minced
- 4 cups chicken broth
- Salt and black pepper, to taste

1. Melt the butter in a large pot over medium heat. Add garlic and cook for one minute until tender. Add mushrooms, salt and pepper, and cook for 10 minutes. Pour the broth over and bring to a boil.
2. Reduce the heat and simmer for 10 minutes. Puree the soup with a hand blender until smooth. Stir in crème fraiche. Garnish with thyme leaves before serving.

PER SERVING

Kcal: 281 | Fat: 25g | Net Carbs: 5.8g | Protein: 6.1g

Mustard Green & Potato Soup

Prep time: 5 minutes | Cook time:25 minutes | Serves 6

- 1 bunch of mustard greens, chopped
- 2 tbsp extra-virgin olive oil
- 1 red onion, chopped
- 1 leek, chopped
- 2 garlic cloves, minced
- 6 cups vegetable broth
- 1 lb sweet potatoes, cubed
- ¼ tsp crushed red pepper

1. Heat the oil in a pot over medium heat.
2. Place onion, leek, and garlic and sauté for 5 minutes.
3. Pour in broth, sweet potatoes, and red pepper.
4. Bring to a boil, then lower the heat and season with salt and pepper.
5. Simmer for 15 minutes.
6. Add in mustard greens, cook for 5 minutes until the greens are tender.
7. Serve and enjoy!

PER SERVING

Cal 140 | Fat 5g | Carbs 23g | Protein 2g

Classic Minestrone Soup

Prep time: 5 minutes | Cook time:15 minutes | Serves 4

- 2 tbsp extra-virgin olive oil
- 1 onion, chopped
- 1 carrot, chopped
- 1 stalk celery, chopped
- 2 garlic cloves, minced
- 4 cups vegetable stock
- 1 cup green peas
- ½ cup orzo
- 1 (15-oz) can diced tomatoes
- 2 tsp Italian seasoning
- Sea salt and pepper to taste

1. Heat the oil in a pot over medium heat.
2. Sauté the onion, garlic, carrot, and celery for 5 minutes until tender.
3. Stir in vegetable stock, green peas, orzo, tomatoes, salt, pepper, and Italian seasoning.
4. Cook for 10 minutes.
5. Serve warm.

PER SERVING

Cal 170| Fat 8g| Carbs 22g| Protein 5g

One-Pot Chunky Beef Stew

Prep time: 5 minutes | Cook time:30 minutes | Serves 6

- 2 tbsp extra-virgin olive oil
- 1 ½ lb sirloin steak, cubed
- 3 chopped sweet potatoes
- 4 baby carrots, sliced
- 1 celery stalk, sliced
- 1 small onion, chopped
- 4 cups beef broth
- 2 garlic cloves, minced
- 1 cup green peas
- ½ tsp dried thyme
- Sea salt and pepper to taste
- 3 tablespoons arrowroot

1. Warm the extra-virgin olive oil in a pot over medium heat.
2. Add the beef, sweet potatoes, baby carrots, celery, garlic, and onion and sauté for 5-8 minutes until the beef is browned.
3. Pour in the broth and thyme.
4. Bring to a boil, lower the heat, and simmer for 15 minutes.
5. Mix the arrowroot with 1 soup ladle in a small bowl and pour the slurry gradually into the pot, whisking continuously.
6. Add the green peas and cook for 2-4 more minutes.
7. Taste and adjust seasoning.
8. Serve warm.

PER SERVING

Cal 396| Fat 13g| Carbs 27.6g| Protein 41g

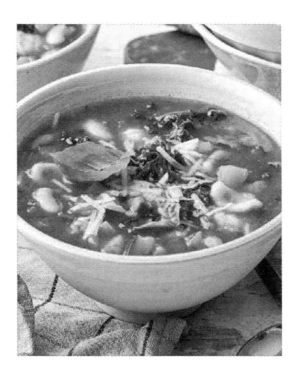

Chapter 11
Salads & Entrées

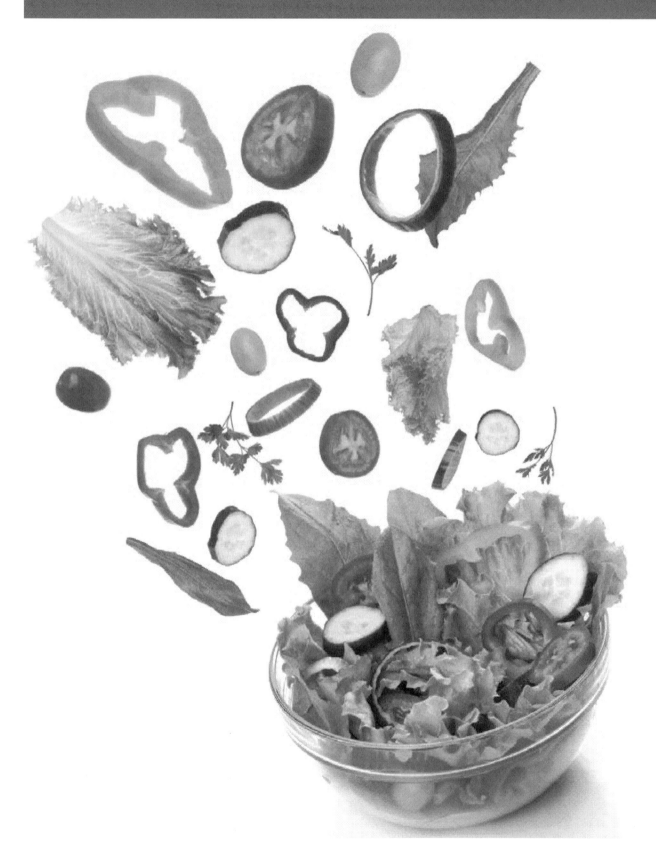

Spinach & Pomegranate Salad

Prep time: 5 minutes | Cook time:5 minutes | Serves 4

- 2 tbsp extra-virgin olive oil
- 4 cups fresh baby spinach
- ¼ cup pomegranate seeds
- ¼ cup raspberry vinaigrette

1. Mix the spinach and walnuts in a bowl.
2. Sprinkle with olive oil and raspberry vinaigrette and toss to combine.

PER SERVING

Cal 500| Fat 49g| Carbs 10g| Protein 12g| Fiber: 5g

Ginger Fruit Salad

Prep time: 5 minutes | Cook time:5 minutes | Serves 4

- 1 nectarine, sliced
- ½ cup fresh blueberries
- ½ cup fresh raspberries
- ½ cup fresh strawberries
- 1 tbsp grated fresh ginger
- 1 orange, zested
- 1 orange, juiced

1. Mix the nectarine, blueberries, raspberries, strawberries, ginger, orange zest, and orange juice in a bowl.
2. Serve.

PER SERVING

Cal 80| Fat 1g| Carbs 19g| Protein 2g| Fiber:4g

Broccoli Salad with Tempeh & Cranberries

Prep time: 5 minutes | Cook time:10 minutes | Serves 4

- 3 oz olive oil
- ¾ lb tempeh slices, cubed
- 1 lb broccoli florets
- Sea salt and pepper to taste
- 2 tbsp almonds, chopped
- ½ cup frozen cranberries

1. In a skillet, warm the olive oil over medium heat until no longer foaming, and fry the tempeh cubes until brown on all sides.
2. Add the broccoli and stir-fry for 6 minutes.
3. Season with salt and pepper.
4. Turn the heat off.
5. Stir in the almonds and cranberries to warm through.
6. Serve.

PER SERVING

Cal 390| Fat 31g| Carbs 13g| Protein 20g| Fiber: 4.4g

Bean & Roasted Parsnip Salad

Prep time: 5 minutes | Cook time:35 minutes | Serves 3

- 1 (15-oz) can cannellini beans
- 4 parsnips, sliced
- 2 tsp olive oil
- ½ tsp ground cinnamon
- Sea salt to taste
- 3 cups chopped spinach
- 2 tsp pomegranate seeds
- 2 tsp sunflower seeds
- ¼ cup raspberry vinaigrette

1. Preheat your oven to 390°F.
2. In a bowl, combine parsnips, olive oil, cinnamon, and salt.
3. Spread on a baking tray and roast for 15 minutes.
4. Flip the parsnips and add the beans.
5. Roast for another 15 minutes.
6. Allow cooling.
7. Divide the spinach among plates and place the pomegranate seeds, sunflower seeds, and roasted parsnips and beans.
8. Sprinkle with raspberry vinaigrette and serve.

PER SERVING

Cal 300| Fat 12g| Carbs 45g| Protein 8g| Fiber:6g

Apple & Kale Salad with Citrus Vinaigrette

Prep time: 5 minutes | Cook time:5 minutes | Serves 2

- 1 cup kale
- ½ apple, cored and chopped
- ¼ red onion, thinly sliced
- 2 tbsp sunflower seeds
- 2 tbsp raisins
- 2 tbsp citrus vinaigrette

1. Place the kale on a plate.
2. Add in apple, red onion, sunflower seeds, and raisins.
3. Sprinkle with vinaigrette and serve.

PER SERVING

Cal 130| Fat 5g| Carbs 22g| Protein 3g| Fiber: 6.4g

Mediterranean Chicken Salads with Tzatziki Sauce

Prep time: 5 minutes | Cook time: 1 hour | Serves 2

CHICKEN:

- 3 tablespoons extra virgin olive oil, divided
- Juice of ½ lemon
- 1 tablespoon organic apple cider vinegar
- ½ teaspoongarlic powder
- 1 pound (about 4) boneless, skinless chicken thighs
- Tzatziki Sauce:
- 1 tablespoon extra virgin olive oil
- ½ cup deseeded andgrated Persian cucumber
- 2garlic cloves, minced
- Juice of 1 lemon
- ¼ teaspoon sea salt

SALAD:

- 3 to 4 cups baby spinach leaves
- ½ cup cherry tomatoes, sliced
- ½ red onion, sliced
- ¼ cup full-fat feta, crumbled
- ¼ cup Kalamata olives, sliced

1. In a small bowl, mix together 2 tablespoons olive oil, lemon juice, cider vinegar, andgarlic powder. Put the chicken thighs in a large bowl and pour the marinade over them. Put the chicken in the refrigerator to marinate for 30 minutes.
2. While the chicken marinates, mix together the tzatziki in a small bowl and set aside.
3. Heat the remaining 1 tablespoon olive oil in a large skillet over medium heat. Add the chicken, cooking the thighs on each side for 8 to 10 minutes, or until cooked through and the internal temperature reaches 165°F.
4. Remove the chicken from the skillet and slice each thigh into four or five pieces.
5. Combine the salad and serve in two bowls, topped with the chicken and tzatziki sauce.

PER SERVING

Calories: 899 | Fat: 67.7g | Saturated Fat: 18.7g | Protein: 61.1g | Carbohydrate: 19.2g | Fiber: 3.2g | Sodium: 1,375mg

Cucumber & Pear Rice Salad

Prep time: 5 minutes | Cook time:10 minutes | Serves 4

- 1 cup brown rice
- ¼ cup olive oil
- ¼ cup orange juice
- 1 pear, cored and diced
- ½ cucumber, diced
- ¼ cup raisins
- Sea salt and pepper to taste

1. Place the rice in a pot with 2 cups of salted water.
2. Bring to a boil, then lower the heat and simmer for 15 minutes.
3. In a bowl, whisk together the olive oil, orange juice, salt, and pepper.
4. Stir in the pear, cucumber, raisins, and cooked rice.
5. Serve.

PER SERVING

Cal 355| Fat 15g| Carbs 52g| Protein 1g| Fiber:5g

Turkey Salad

Prep time: 5 minutes | Cook time: 10 minutes | Serves 4

- 1 pound turkey breast, cooked
- 3green onions, sliced
- 2 celery stalks, diced
- ½ cup chopped walnuts
- ½ cup avocado oil mayonnaise
- 1 teaspoon fresh lemon juice
- ¼ teaspoon sea salt
- ¼ teaspoon freshlyground black pepper
- Mixedgreens

1. Chop the turkey breast into small pieces.
2. In a large bowl, combine the turkey, onions, celery, walnuts, mayonnaise, lemon juice, salt, and pepper, and mix well.
3. Serve on a bed of mixedgreens.

PER SERVING

Calories: 351 | Fat: 22.8g | Saturated Fat: 2.2g | Protein: 31.8g | Carbohydrate: 5.4g | Fiber: 2g | Sodium: 254mg

Fantastic Spinach & Chicken Salad

Prep time: 5 minutes | Cook time:20 minutes | Serves 2

- 1 chicken breasts, chopped
- 1 carrot, sliced
- 1 tbsp extra-virgin olive oil
- 1 shallot, chopped
- 1 tsp ground cumin
- ½ avocado, chopped
- 1 lime, juiced
- ½ cucumber, chopped
- ½ cup baby spinach

1. Warm the oil in the pan over medium heat and sauté the chicken for 8-10 minutes until browned and cooked through.
2. Remove and let it cool.
3. To the same pan, add the carrot and shallot and continue to cook for 5 minutes.
4. Season with cumin.
5. Mash the avocado and lime juice with a fork.
6. Layer a jar with half of the avocado mixture, then the cumin roasted veggies, and then the chicken, packing it all in.
7. Top with cucumbers, cilantro, and baby spinach.
8. Chill in the fridge before serving.

PER SERVING

Cal 520| Fat 23g| Carbs 17g| Protein 63g| Fiber: 4.4g

African Zucchini Salad
Prep time: 5 minutes | Cook time:15 minutes | Serves 2

- 1 lemon, half zested and juiced, half cut into wedges
- 1 tsp olive oil
- 1 zucchini, chopped
- ½ tsp ground cumin
- ½ tsp ground ginger
- ¼ tsp turmeric
- ¼ tsp ground nutmeg
- A pinch of sea salt
- 2 tbsp capers
- 1 tbsp chopped green olives
- 1 garlic clove, pressed
- 2 tbsp fresh mint, chopped
- 2 cups spinach, chopped

1. Warm the olive oil in a skillet over medium heat.
2. Place the zucchini and sauté for 10 minutes.
3. Stir in cumin, ginger, turmeric, nutmeg, and salt.
4. Pour in lemon zest, lemon juice, capers, garlic, and mint and cook for 2 minutes more.
5. Divide the spinach between serving plates and top with zucchini mixture.
6. Garnish with lemon and olives.

PER SERVING

Cal 50| Fat 3g| Carbs 5g| Protein 41| Fiber: 8g

Drop-The-Chopstick Bowl
Prep time: 5 minutes | Cook time: 26 minutes | Serves 5

- 2 tablespoons sesame oil
- 2 cloves garlic, peeled and minced
- 1 pound lean ground beef
- 1 (14-ounce) bag coleslaw mix
- 1 tablespoon sriracha sauce
- 1 tablespoon white vinegar
- 2 tablespoons soy sauce
- ⅛ teaspoon salt
- ⅛ teaspoon black pepper
- 1 teaspoon sesame seeds
- 1 medium green onion, finely chopped

1. In a large skillet over medium heat, heat oil. Add garlic and sauté 1 minute, then add ground beef. Fully cook meat until all pink is gone, approximately 15 minutes. Drain fat.
2. Thoroughly stir in coleslaw mix, sriracha sauce, vinegar, and soy sauce. Cook 10 minutes while stirring until coleslaw is wilted.
3. Season with salt and pepper and garnish with sesame seeds and green onion sprinkled on top.

PER SERVING

Calories: 280 | Fat: 15g | Protein: 24g | Sodium: 673mg| Fiber: 3g |Carbohydrates: 8g | Net Carbs: 5g | Sugar: 4g

Mediterranean Pasta Salad
Prep time: 5 minutes | Cook time:10 minutes | Serves 4

- ½ cup minced sun-dried tomatoes
- 2 roasted bell red peppers, chopped
- 8 oz whole-wheat pasta
- 1 (15.5-oz) can chickpeas
- ½ cup pitted black olives
- 1 (6-oz) jar dill pickles, sliced
- ½ cup frozen peas, thawed
- 1 tbsp capers
- 3 tsp dried chives
- ½ cup olive oil
- ¼ cup white wine vinegar
- ½ tsp dried basil
- 1 garlic clove, minced
- Sea salt and pepper to taste

1. Cook the pasta in salted water for 8-10 minutes until al dente.
2. Drain and remove to a bowl.
3. Stir in chickpeas, black olives, sun-dried tomatoes, dill pickles, roasted peppers, peas, capers, and chives.
4. In another bowl, whisk oil, white wine vinegar, basil, garlic, sugar, salt, and pepper.
5. Pour over the pasta and toss to coat.
6. Serve.

PER SERVING

Cal 590| Fat 32g| Carbs 67g| Protein 12g| Fiber: 4.4g

Mushroom and Green Bean Salad
Prep time: 5 minutes | Cook time:20 minutes | Serves 4

- 1 lb cremini mushrooms, sliced
- ½ cup green beans
- 3 tbsp olive oil
- Sea salt and pepper to taste
- Juice of 1 lemon
- 4 tbsp toasted hazelnuts

1. Preheat your oven to 450°F.
2. Arrange the mushrooms and green beans in a baking dish, drizzle the olive oil over, and sprinkle with salt and black pepper.
3. Use your hands to rub the vegetables with the seasoning and roast in the oven for 20 minutes or until they are soft.
4. Transfer the vegetables into a salad bowl, drizzle with the lemon juice, and toss the salad with hazelnuts.
5. Serve and enjoy!

PER SERVING

Cal 130| Fat 11g| Carbs 6g| Protein 11g| Fiber: 6.4g

Caprese Salad

Prep time: 5 minutes | Cook time: 10 minutes | Serves 8

- 8 ounces fresh mozzarella cheese
- 4 tomatoes
- ¼ cup balsamic vinegar
- ¼ cup extra virgin olive oil
- 1 cup fresh basil
- 1 teaspoon sea salt
- ½ teaspoon freshlyground black pepper

1. Cut the mozzarella and tomatoes into ¼-inch-thick slices and arrange in an alternating pattern on a plate.
2. In a small bowl, mix the balsamic vinegar and olive oil. Drizzle on top of the mozzarella and tomatoes.
3. Stack the fresh basil and roll it into a tight log. Carefully cut into thin julienne slices, and toss over the salad.
4. Sprinkle the salt and pepper on top and enjoy.

PER SERVING

Calories: 148 | Fat: 11.4g | Saturated Fat: 3.9g | Protein: 8.6g | Carbohydrate: 3.6g | Fiber: 0.8g | Sodium: 408mg

Egg Tahini Salad

Prep time: 5 minutes | Cook time: 5 minutes | Serves 4

- 3 cups freshgreens
- 2 Roma tomatoes, diced
- 1 bell pepper, diced
- ½ cup sliced radishes
- 1 avocado, sliced
- 6 hard-boiled eggs
- 2 ounces Tahini Lemon Dressing

1. In a large bowl, combine thegreens, tomatoes, bell pepper, radishes, and avocado.
2. Slice, chop, or quarter the eggs and place them on top of the salad.
3. Drizzle with the dressing and serve in individual bowls.

PER SERVING

Calories: 355 | Fat: 28.3g | Saturated Fat: 5.8g | Protein: 13.4g | Carbohydrate: 16.8g | Fiber: 7.6g | Sodium: 121mg

Vintage Three Bean Salad

Prep time: 15 minutes | Cook time: 5 minutes | Serves 4

- 3 cups fresh green beans, trimmed and cut into 2" lengths
- ½ cup shelled soybeans (edamame), cooked
- 1 cup black soybeans
- 3 tablespoons olive oil
- 2 tablespoons apple cider vinegar
- 1 tablespoon lemon juice
- 1 teaspoon spicy mustard
- 1 clove garlic, peeled and minced
- 2 tablespoons dried basil, or chopped fresh
- ⅛ teaspoon salt
- ⅛ teaspoon black pepper

1. In a medium microwave-safe bowl, microwave raw green beans 4 minutes with ¼ cup water. Drain water and let cool.
2. In a medium mixing bowl, combine green beans with other two beans.
3. In a small bowl, whisk remaining ingredients to make dressing.
4. Pour dressing over beans and lightly toss.
5. If desired, chill before serving.

PER SERVING

Calories: 204 | Fat: 14g | Protein: 10g | Sodium: 111mg | Fiber: 7g | Carbohydrates: 13g | Net Carbs: 6g | Sugar: 3g

Thai Green Bean & Mango Salad

Prep time: 5 minutes | Cook time:10 minutes | Serves 4

- 1 mango, julienned
- 8 oz green beans, trimmed
- ½ cup chopped mint
- ½ cup chopped cilantro
- ½ cup chopped almonds
- 12 cherry tomatoes, halved
- 2 red Thai chiles, sliced
- 3 tbsp sugar-free soy sauce
- 2 tbsp raw honey
- ½ cup lime juice

1. Steam the green beans for approximately 2 minutes or until crisp-tender.
2. Drain and slice them in half crosswise.
3. Combine red chilies, soy sauce, honey, and lime juice in a bowl and stir well.
4. Combine the green beans with the remaining ingredients in a large serving bowl.
5. Drizzle with the dressing, then toss to combine well.
6. Serve.

PER SERVING

Cal 155| Fat 1g| Carbs 37g| Protein 5g| Fiber: 6.4g

Buffalo Chili

Prep time: 5 minutes | Cook time: 1 hour, 20 minutes | Serves 8

- 1 tablespoon coconut oil
- 2 poundsground bison meat
- 1 large poblano pepper, diced
- ½ large onion, diced
- 3garlic cloves, minced
- 1 (15-ounce) can roasted tomatoes
- 1 (15-ounce) can tomato sauce (no sugar added)
- 1 cup beef broth
- ¼ cup chili powder
- 1 tablespoonground cumin
- 1 teaspoon sea salt
- Toppings (optional):
- Avocado
- Grass-fed shredded cheese
- Sour cream

1. Heat the coconut oil in a large stockpot over medium heat. Add the bison meat and cook for 8 to 10 minutes, or until browned.
2. Add the pepper, onion, andgarlic to the pot. Stir well and cook for 10 minutes. Stir in the tomatoes, tomato sauce, and broth. Add the chili powder, cumin, and salt.
3. Bring to a boil, stir well, reduce the heat to low, and cover. Let it simmer for about 1 hour, stirring occasionally.
4. Serve in bowls with the toppings (if using).

PER SERVING

Calories: 192 | Fat: 10.8g | Saturated Fat: 5g | Protein: 11.3g | Carbohydrate: 14.2g | Fiber: 4.7g | Sodium: 1,069mg

Olive Garden Salad

Prep time: 10 minutes | Cook time: 5 minutes | Serves 4

- 6 cups chopped iceberg lettuce
- 2 Roma tomatoes, sliced into rounds
- ¼ cup sliced red onion
- 1 cup whole pepperoncini
- 1 cup whole black olives
- 3 tablespoons olive oil
- 1 tablespoon red wine vinegar
- ¼ teaspoon garlic powder
- ⅛ teaspoon salt
- ⅛ teaspoon black pepper
- ⅓ cup grated Parmesan cheese

1. Mix all vegetables and olives in a large salad bowl.
2. In a small bowl, mix oil, vinegar, and spices together.
3. Pour dressing over salad, toss, and top with Parmesan cheese. Serve immediately.

PER SERVING

Calories: 217 | Fat: 18g | Protein: 4g | Sodium: 948mg| Fiber: 2g |Carbohydrates: 8g | Net Carbs: 6g | Sugar: 3g

Summer Tuna Avocado Salad

Prep time: 10 minutes | Cook time: 5 minutes | Serves 4

- 3 (5-ounce) cans tuna in water, drained and flaked
- 1 medium cucumber, sliced
- 3 medium avocados, peeled, pitted, and sliced
- 1 medium red onion, peeled and sliced
- ¼ cup finely chopped cilantro
- 2 tablespoons lemon juice
- 2 tablespoons olive oil
- ⅛ teaspoon salt
- ⅛ teaspoon black pepper

1. In a medium mixing bowl, add drained, flaked tuna.
2. Lightly toss cucumber, avocados, onion, cilantro, lemon juice, and olive oil with tuna. Lightly add salt and pepper at end.
3. Serve immediately.

PER SERVING

Calories: 362 | Fat: 23g | Protein: 23g | Sodium: 403mg| Fiber: 8g |Carbohydrates: 15g | Net Carbs: 7g | Sugar: 3g

Big Mac Salad

Prep time: 10 minutes | Cook time: 15 minutes | Serves 4

- 1 pound lean ground turkey
- 6 cups chopped iceberg lettuce
- 1 large pickle, sliced into thin rounds
- ½ cup diced onion
- ½ cup diced tomato
- ⅓ cup shredded Cheddar cheese
- 1 tablespoon sesame seeds
- ¼ cup full-fat mayonnaise
- ¼ cup no-sugar-added ketchup

1. In a medium skillet over medium heat, cook ground turkey until well done (about 10–15 minutes), stirring regularly. Do not drain fat. Let cool.
2. In a large salad bowl, toss lettuce, pickle, onion, tomato, and shredded cheese.
3. Stir in cooled meat.
4. In a small bowl, mix the sauce ingredients. Add to salad and toss.
5. Sprinkle salad with sesame seeds and serve.

PER SERVING

Calories: 347 | Fat: 23g | Protein: 25g | Sodium: 699mg| Fiber: 2g |Carbohydrates: 8g | Net Carbs: 6g | Sugar: 5g

Chapter 12
Desserts

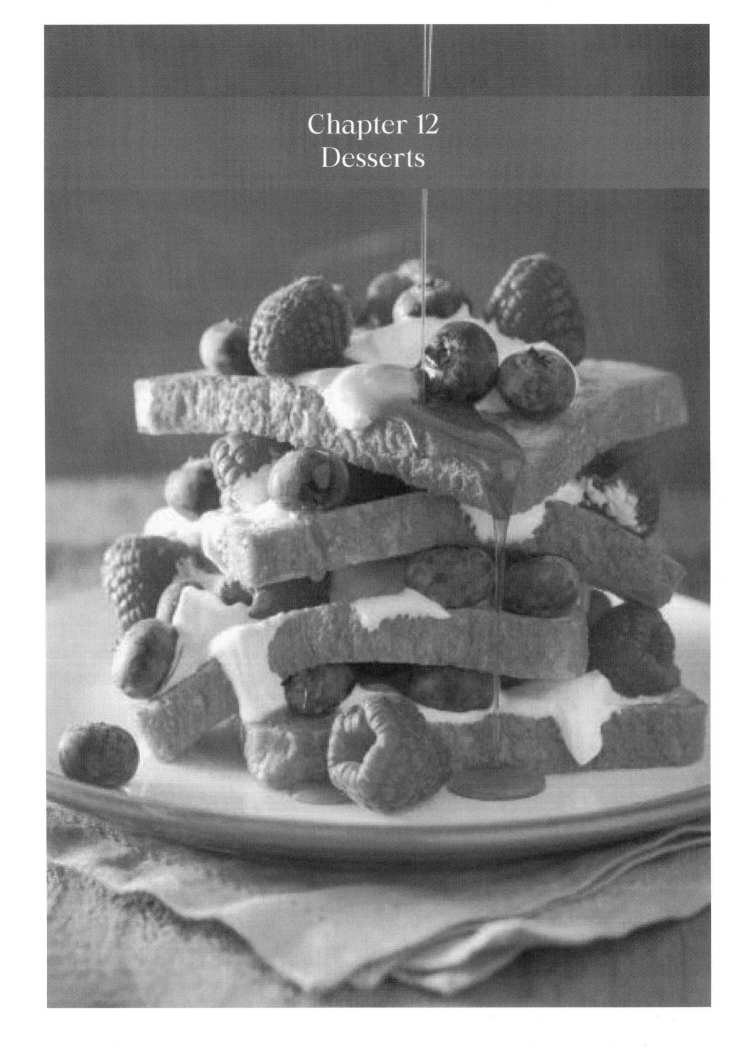

Apple-Cinnamon Compote

Prep time: 5 minutes | Cook time: 20minutes | Serves 4

- 6 peeled apples, chopped
- 1 tsp fresh lemon juice
- ¼ cup orange juice
- ¼ cup honey
- 1 tsp ground cinnamon
- A pinch of sea salt

1. Place the apples, orange juice, lemon juice, honey, cinnamon, and salt in a pot over medium heat and simmer for 10 minutes until the apples are tender.
2. Let cool completely before serving.

PER SERVING

Cal 250| Fat 1g| Carbs 67g| Protein 8g

Greek Cheesecake with Blueberries

Prep time: 5 minutes | Cook time: 85minutes | Serves 6

- 2 oz almond butter
- 1¼ cups almond flour
- 3 tbsp stevia
- 1 tsp vanilla extract
- 3 eggs
- 2 cups Greek yogurt
- ½ cup coconut cream
- 1 tsp lemon zest
- 2 oz fresh blueberries

1. Preheat oven to 350°F.
2. To make the crust, put the almond butter in a skillet over low heat until nutty in flavor.
3. Turn the heat off and stir in almond flour, 2 tbsp of stevia, and half of vanilla until a dough forms.
4. Press the mixture into a greased baking pan.
5. Bake for 8 minutes.
6. In a bowl, combine yogurt, coconut cream, remaining stevia, lemon zest, remaining vanilla extract, and eggs.
7. Remove the crust from the oven and pour the mixture on top.
8. Use a spatula to layer evenly.
9. Bake the cake for 15 minutes at 400°F.
10. Cool completely.
11. Refrigerate overnight and scatter the blueberries on top.
12. Serve.

PER SERVING

Cal 425| Fat 40g| Carbs 12g| Protein 8g

Party Matcha & Hazelnut Cheesecake

Prep time: 5 minutes | Cook time: 15 minutes | Serves 4

- 2 tbsp toasted hazelnuts, chopped
- 2/3 cup toasted rolled oats
- ¼ cup almond butter, melted
- 3 tbsp pure date sugar
- 6 oz coconut cream
- ¼ cup almond milk
- 1 tbsp matcha powder
- ¼ cup just-boiled water
- 3 tsp agar agar powder

1. Process the oats, butter, and date sugar in a blender until smooth.
2. Pour the mixture into a greased springform pan and press the mixture onto the bottom of the pan.
3. Refrigerate for 30 minutes until firm while you make the filling.
4. In a large bowl, using an electric mixer, whisk the coconut cream cheese until smooth.
5. Beat in the almond milk and mix in the matcha powder until smooth.
6. Mix the boiled water and agar agar until dissolved and whisk this mixture into the creamy mix.
7. Fold in the hazelnuts until well distributed.
8. Remove the cake pan from the fridge and pour in the cream mixture.
9. Shake the pan to ensure smooth layering on top.
10. Refrigerate further for at least 3 hours.
11. Take out the cake pan, release the cake, slice, and serve.

PER SERVING

Cal 650| Fat 59g| Carbs 26g| Protein 14g

"Frosty" Chocolate Shake

Prep time: 10 minutes | Cook time: 5 minutes | Serves 2

- 1 cup heavy (whipping) cream or coconut cream
- 2 tablespoons unsweetened cocoa powder
- 1 tablespoon almond butter
- 1 teaspoon vanilla extract
- 5 or 6 drops liquid stevia

1. In a medium bowl or using a stand mixer, beat the cream until fluffy, 3 to 4 minutes.
2. Add the cocoa powder, almond butter, vanilla, and stevia. Beat the mixture for an additional 2 to 3 minutes, or until the mixture has the consistency of whipped cream.
3. Place the bowl in the freezer for 25 to 30 minutes before serving.

PER SERVING

Calories: 493 | Fat: 49g | Protein: 5g | Total Carbs: 8g | Net Carbs: 5g | Fiber: 3g | Sugar: 1g | Sodium: 47mg | Macros: Fat: 89% | Protein: 4% | Carbs: 7%

Nutty Chocolate Biscotti

Prep time: 20 minutes | Cooking time: 1 hour | Serves 12

- For The Biscotti:
- 2 tablespoons flaxseed meal (ground flax seeds)
- 6 tablespoons water
- 2 cups almond flour, sifted for best results
- ½ cup sunflower seeds, ground into a flour
- 1 teaspoon baking powder
- ⅓ cup pecans or walnuts, chopped
- Zest of 1 lemon and 1 orange
- 3 tablespoons stevia powder extract
- 1 teaspoon pure almond extract
- For The Chocolate Glaze:
- 2 tablespoons finely chopped/shaved bakers' chocolate (100 percent cocoa, no sugar)
- ¼ cup monk fruit sweetener
- 1½ tablespoons virgin coconut oil

1. Preheat oven to 300°F with the oven rack set in the middle. Prepare the flax egg by mixing the flax meal and water in a small bowl and allow to sit at least 15 minutes so it can thicken.
2. Sift the almond flour in a large bowl. Use a coffee grinder or food processor to turn the sunflower seeds into flour. To the almond flour, add the ground sunflower seeds, baking powder, lemon and orange zest, and pecans, and mix well with a whisk.
3. Pour the flax seed egg mixture into a separate bowl and add the stevia powder, almond extract, and coconut oil, and mix well. Add the wet batter on top of the dry batter and mix well until the dough comes together. Use your hands to mix once the dough firms up.
4. Place a piece of parchment paper on a sheet tray and use your hands and form the dough into a ten-by-three-inch log. You can make the shape wider and shorter if desired. Bake for 35 minutes, then remove from oven and allow to cool down for 15 minutes.
5. Once cooled, use a sharp knife to cut the log into ¾-inch biscotti pieces and lay them on a cooling rack. Place the cooling rack on the sheet pan and bake for another 25–30 minutes until the biscotti are golden brown and have color around the edges. If you don't have a cooling rack, flip the biscotti halfway to ensure even baking on each side.

FOR THE CHOCOLATE GLAZE

1. Prepare a double boiler or use the microwave to melt the chocolate. Once the chocolate is melted, add the monk fruit sweetener and coconut oil and whisk until the sauce is smooth and creamy. If it is a bit grainy or cools down before drizzling, continue heating until smooth.
2. Remove biscotti from oven and allow to cool for 10 minutes before drizzling with chocolate sauce. Enjoy!

PER SERVING

Calories: 131 | Fat: 8g | Protein: 3g | Total Carbs: 13g | Fiber: 1g | Sugar: 5g | Sodium: 32mg | Protein: 9% | Carbs: 40%

Pistachios & Chocolate Popsicles

Prep time: 5 minutes | Cook time:5 minutes | Serves 4

- 2 oz dark chocolate, melted
- 1½ cups oat milk
- 1 tbsp cocoa powder
- 3 tbsp pure date syrup
- 1 tsp vanilla extract
- 2 tbsp pistachios, chopped

1. In a blender, add chocolate, oat milk, cocoa powder, date syrup, vanilla, pistachios, and process until smooth.
2. Divide the mixture into popsicle molds and freeze for 3 hours.
3. Dip the popsicle molds in warm water to loosen the popsicles and pull out the popsicles.

PER SERVING

Cal 120| Fat 3g| Carbs 24g| Protein 6g | Fiber: 5g

Coconut Chocolate Truffles

Prep time: 5 minutes | Cook time: 70 minutes | Serves 6

- 1 cup raw cashews, soaked
- ¾ cup pitted cherries
- 2 tbsp coconut oil
- 1 cup shredded coconut
- 2 tbsp cocoa powder

1. Line a baking sheet with parchment paper and set aside.
2. Blend cashews, cherries, coconut oil, half of the shredded coconut, and cocoa powder in a food processor until ingredients are evenly mixed.
3. Spread the remaining shredded coconut on a dish.
4. Mold the mixture into 12 truffle shapes.
5. Roll the truffles in the coconut dish, shaking off any excess, then arrange on the prepared baking sheet.
6. Refrigerate for 1 hour.
7. Serve and enjoy!

PER SERVING

Cal 320| Fat 28g| Carbs 18g| Protein 6g

Oatmeal Cookies with Hazelnuts

Prep time: 5 minutes | Cook time:10 minutes | Serves 2

- 1 ½ cups whole-grain flour
- 1 tsp baking powder
- 1 tsp ground cinnamon
- ¼ tsp ground nutmeg
- 1 ½ cups old-fashioned oats
- 1 cup chopped hazelnuts
- ½ cup almond butter, melted
- ½ cup pure maple syrup
- ¼ cup pure date sugar
- 2 tsp pure vanilla extract

1. Preheat your oven to 360°F.
2. Combine the flour, baking powder, cinnamon, and nutmeg in a bowl.
3. Add in oats and hazelnuts.
4. In another bowl, whisk the almond butter, maple syrup, sugar, and vanilla.
5. Pour over the flour mixture.
6. Mix.
7. Spoon a small ball of cookie dough on a baking sheet and press down with a fork.
8. Bake for 10-12 minutes until browned.
9. Let completely cool on a rack.

PER SERVING

Cal 1580| Fat 95g| Carbs 190g| Protein 35g

Cookies And Cream Parfait

Prep time: 5 minutes | Cook time:5 minutes |Serves 1

- ½ scoop low-carb vanilla protein powder
- ¾ cup plain full-fat Greek yogurt
- 1 Oreo cookie
- 4 tablespoons sugar-free chocolate syrup (I like Walden Farms)

1. In a small bowl, mix together the protein powder and Greek yogurt until smooth and creamy.
2. Remove one side of the Oreo cookie. Place it in a small resealable plastic bag and crush it with the back of a spoon. Set aside.
3. Pour the chocolate syrup over the yogurt mixture and sprinkle with the cookie crumbles.

PER SERVING

Calories: 281 | Fat: 13g | Protein: 19g | Total Carbs: 22g | Net Carbs: 19g | Fiber: 3g | Sugar: 16g | Sodium: 236mg | Macros: Fat: 42% | Protein: 27% | Carbs: 31%

Pecan Pie Pudding

Prep time: 5 minutes | Cook time:5 minutes |Serves 1

- ¾ cup plain full-fat Greek yogurt
- ½ scoop low-carb vanilla protein powder
- 4 tablespoons chopped pecans
- 2 tablespoons sugar-free syrup

1. In a small bowl, mix together the Greek yogurt and protein powder until smooth and creamy.
2. Top with the chopped pecans and syrup.

PER SERVING

Calories: 381 | Fat: 21g | Protein: 32g | Total Carbs: 16g | Net Carbs: 9g | Fiber: 7g | Sugar: 6g | Sodium: 143mg | Macros: Fat: 50% | Protein: 34% | Carbs: 16%

Chocolate Avocado Pudding

Prep time: 5 minutes | Cook time:5 minutes |Serves 1

- 1 avocado, halved
- ⅓ cup full-fat coconut milk
- 1 teaspoon vanilla extract
- 2 tablespoons unsweetened cocoa powder
- 5 or 6 drops liquid stevia

1. Combine all the ingredients in a high-powered blender or food processor and blend until smooth. Serve immediately.

PER SERVING

Calories: 555 | Fat: 47g | Protein: 7g | Total Carbs: 26g | Fiber: 17g | Sugar: 4g | Sodium: 29mg | Protein: 5% | Carbs: 19%

Coconut & Chocolate Macaroons

Prep time: 5 minutes | Cook time:20 minutes | Serves 4

- 1 cup shredded coconut
- 2 tbsp cocoa powder
- 1 tbsp vanilla extract
- 1 cup coconut milk
- ¼ cup maple syrup
- A pinch of salt

1. Preheat your oven to 360°F.
2. Place the shredded coconut, cocoa powder, vanilla extract, coconut milk, maple syrup, and salt in a pot.
3. Cook until a firm dough is formed.
4. Shape balls out of the mixture.
5. Arrange the balls on a lined with parchment paper baking sheet.
6. Bake for 15 minutes.
7. Allow cooling before serving.

PER SERVING

Cal 170| Fat 10g| Carbs 20g| Protein 2g

Pressure Cooked Cherry Pie

Prep time: 5 minutes | Cook time:40minutes | Serves 6

- 1 9-inch double pie crust
- ½ tsp vanilla extract
- 4 cups cherries, pitted
- ¼ tsp almond extract
- 4 tbsp quick tapioca
- 1 cup packed brown sugar
- A pinch of sea salt

1. Add 1 cup of water to the Instant Pot and place the steam rack on top.
2. Combine the cherries with tapioca, sugar, extracts, and salt.
3. Place one pie crust on the bottom of a lined springform pan.
4. Spread the filling over.
5. Top with the other crust.
6. Place the pan on the steam rack.
7. Seal the lid and cook for 18 minutes on "Manual" on high pressure.
8. Wait 10 minutes before releasing the pressure quickly.
9. Carefully remove the top so that any condensation doesn't drip on the pie, then carefully remove the pan using oven mitts or tongs.
10. Let it cool for at least 5 minutes before serving.

PER SERVING

Cal 395| Fat 12g| Carbs 70g| Protein 2g | Fiber: 10g

Mango Chocolate Fudge

Prep time: 5 minutes | Cook time:5 minutes | Serves 3

- 1 mango, pureed
- ¾ cup dark chocolate chips
- 4 cups pure date sugar

1. Microwave the chocolate until melted.
2. Add in the pureed mango and date sugar and stir to combine.
3. Spread on a lined with waxed paper baking pan and chill in the fridge for 2 hours.
4. Take out the fudge and lay on a cutting board.
5. Slice into small pieces and serve.

PER SERVING

Calories: 109 | Fat: 9g | Protein: 2g | Total Carbs: 10g | Fiber: 2g | Sugar: 6g | Sodium: 1mg | Protein: 7% | Carbs: 36% | Fat: 57%

The Best Keto Fat Bread

Prep time: 15 minutes | Cooking time: 40 minutes | Serves 1 loaf of bread

- 1 cup macadamia nuts unsalted, and roasted if desired
- 5 good quality eggs
- ½ teaspoon kosher salt
- Zest of ½ lemon
- 1 teaspoon baking soda
- 1 tablespoon fresh lemon juice
- 1 cup softened coconut butter (manna)
- 1 teaspoon baking powder
- 1-2 tablespoons everything bagel seasoning

1. Preheat oven to 350°F and make sure the oven rack is set in the middle. Add the macadamia nuts to a food processor or a powerful blender and process for about 30 seconds on high until almost creamy. While the machine is running, add the eggs one at a time, making sure each one has been incorporated into the batter before adding the next one. Turn the machine off and add the salt, lemon zest, baking soda, and add the lemon juice on top of the baking soda to activate it. Turn the machine on and process for another 15 seconds. Turn the machine off and add the softened coconut butter/manna (you can soften it a microwave or in warm water) and process until smooth and creamy. Turn the machine off and add the baking powder and process for 15-20 seconds. It's important to add the baking powder at the end (not when you're adding the baking soda and lemon juice, as that will change the texture of your bread).
2. Line the inside of a non-stick 10 x 4.5-inch bread or meatloaf tin with parchment paper. If you don't have parchment paper, rub the inside with coconut or avocado oil or spray with a cooking spray. Pour the batter into the tin and tap it on the counter a couple times. Sprinkle on the everything bagel seasoning and use your fingers to gently press it down into the batter, so it does not fall off. Bake in the oven for 40-45 minutes or until nicely golden brown on top. Remove from oven, allow to sit in tin for 5 minutes, and then lift bread out using the parchment paper and transfer to a cooling rack for 15 minutes.
3. Slice the bread and enjoy!

PER SERVING

Calories: 193 | Fat: 16g | Protein: 6g | Total Carbs: 6g | Fiber: 3g | Net Carbs: 3g | Sugar: 0g | Sodium: 212mg | Cholesterol: 74mg

Game Day Guacamole

Prep time: 10 minutes | Cooking time: 10 minutes | Serves 4

- ¼ cup finely chopped red onions
- 1–2 limes
- 1 poblano pepper
- 2 tablespoons pepitas
- ½ teaspoon cumin
- 2 large ripe avocados
- 1 teaspoon extra virgin olive oil
- ¼ cup tomatoes, seeds removed and chopped
- Freshly chopped cilantro or parsley
- Kosher salt

1. Add the chopped red onions to a small bowl and squeeze over enough lime juice to cover. Allow it to sit for 10–30 minutes. Place the poblano pepper directly on the stovetop burner set to medium-high and char on all sides for about 10 minutes. Remove and place in a bowl and cover with plastic wrap for 5–10 minutes. Then peel away the charred skin, remove the seeds, and finely chop.
2. Toast the pepitas (Mexican pumpkin seeds) in a non-stick pan with a shot of oil, a pinch of salt, and ½ teaspoon of cumin. Cook over medium heat until golden brown, about 6 minutes. Remove and roughly chop.
3. Scoop the avocados into a bowl. Add ¼ teaspoon of salt and 1 teaspoon extra virgin olive oil. Next, use a potato masher or large fork to mash to desired consistency. I like it chunky. Add the strained red onions, saving the lime juice, chopped tomatoes, pepitas, poblano pepper, 1–2 teaspoons chopped cilantro, and mix well. Check for seasoning as you may need more salt and reserved lime juice from the red onions.

PER SERVING

Calories: 170 | Fat: 15g | Protein: 2g | Total Carbs: 9g | Fiber: 6g | Sugar: 1g | Sodium: 198mg | Protein: 5% | Carbs: 27%

Soft And Cheesy Pita Bread

Prep time: 15 minutes | Cooking time: 15 minutes | Serves 5 pita breads

- 2 eggs
- 2 teaspoons baking powder
- ½ teaspoon kosher salt
- 2 cups or 6 ounces by weight of finely shredded full-fat mozzarella cheese
- 1½ cups blanched almond flour
- ½ teaspoon dried thyme

1. Preheat oven to 400°F. In a large bowl, beat the eggs, add the salt and baking powder, and mix well. Add the finely grated cheese and mix well with a spatula. Add the almond flour and mix well. Put some oil on your hands and continue mixing with your hands.
2. Then separate the dough into five equal balls. Flatten each ball and spread them out on a piece of parchment paper. Next, place another piece of parchment paper on top of the flattened dough. Use a rolling pin to flatten each ball until they are about 5–6 inches in diameter. It's ok if the edges are touching each other.
3. Transfer the dough and bottom piece of parchment to a sheet tray, sprinkle with dried thyme, and bake for 13–15 minutes or until golden brown. Remove from the oven, allow to cool for 5–10 minutes, and enjoy.

PER SERVING

Calories: 187 | Fat: 4g | Protein: 6g | Total Carbs: 32g | Fiber: 2g | Sugar: 1g | Sodium: 337mg | Protein: 13% | Carbs: 68% | Fat: 19%

Appendix 1 Measurement Conversion Chart

Volume Equivalents (Dry)

US STANDARD	METRIC (APPROXIMATE)
1/8 teaspoon	0.5 mL
1/4 teaspoon	1 mL
1/2 teaspoon	2 mL
3/4 teaspoon	4 mL
1 teaspoon	5 mL
1 tablespoon	15 mL
1/4 cup	59 mL
1/2 cup	118 mL
3/4 cup	177 mL
1 cup	235 mL
2 cups	475 mL
3 cups	700 mL
4 cups	1 L

Weight Equivalents

US STANDARD	METRIC (APPROXIMATE)
1 ounce	28 g
2 ounces	57 g
5 ounces	142 g
10 ounces	284 g
15 ounces	425 g
16 ounces (1 pound)	455 g
1.5 pounds	680 g
2 pounds	907 g

Volume Equivalents (Liquid)

US STANDARD	US STANDARD (OUNCES)	METRIC (APPROXIMATE)
2 tablespoons	1 fl.oz.	30 mL
1/4 cup	2 fl.oz.	60 mL
1/2 cup	4 fl.oz.	120 mL
1 cup	8 fl.oz.	240 mL
1 1/2 cup	12 fl.oz.	355 mL
2 cups or 1 pint	16 fl.oz.	475 mL
4 cups or 1 quart	32 fl.oz.	1 L
1 gallon	128 fl.oz.	4 L

Temperatures Equivalents

FAHRENHEIT(F)	CELSIUS(C) APPROXIMATE
225 °F	107 °C
250 °F	120 ° °C
275 °F	135 °C
300 °F	150 °C
325 °F	160 °C
350 °F	180 °C
375 °F	190 °C
400 °F	205 °C
425 °F	220 °C
450 °F	235 °C
475 °F	245 °C
500 °F	260 °C

Appendix 2 The Dirty Dozen and Clean Fifteen

The Environmental Working Group (EWG) is a nonprofit, nonpartisan organization dedicated to protecting human health and the environment Its mission is to empower people to live healthier lives in a healthier environment. This organization publishes an annual list of the twelve kinds of produce, in sequence, that have the highest amount of pesticide residue-the Dirty Dozen-as well as a list of the fifteen kinds ofproduce that have the least amount of pesticide residue-the Clean Fifteen.

THE DIRTY DOZEN	
The 2016 Dirty Dozen includes the following produce. These are considered among the year's most important produce to buy organic:	
Strawberries	Spinach
Apples	Tomatoes
Nectarines	Bell peppers
Peaches	Cherry tomatoes
Celery	Cucumbers
Grapes	Kale/collard greens
Cherries	Hot peppers

The Dirty Dozen list contains two additional itemskale/collard greens and hot peppers-because they tend to contain trace levels of highly hazardous pesticides.

THE CLEAN FIFTEEN	
The least critical to buy organically are the Clean Fifteen list. The following are on the 2016 list:	
Avocados	Papayas
Corn	Kiw
Pineapples	Eggplant
Cabbage	Honeydew
Sweet peas	Grapefruit
Onions	Cantaloupe
Asparagus	Cauliflower
Mangos	

Some of the sweet corn sold in the United States are made from genetically engineered (GE) seedstock. Buy organic varieties of these crops to avoid GE produce.

Appendix 3 Index

COLLEEN L. MCGEE

Made in the USA
Coppell, TX
10 August 2023

20190243R00057